PRAISE FOR
So Heavy a Weight

"*So Heavy a Weight* is a needed contribution to the near-nonexistent canon on reproductive health. I learned more in this collection than I did in all of school plus adulthood. This is required reading for everyone, and it's also great reading."
—Elissa Bassist, author of *Hysterical*

"Every story boldly tells of life, raw and intimate. The collection inspires empathy, validates experiences, and empowers readers to lend their own voices to a collective truth that must be heard."
—Abby Norman, author of *Ask Me About My Uterus: A Quest to Make Doctors Believe in Women's Pain*

"*So Heavy a Weight* is a timely and vital contribution to the ongoing conversation surrounding women's reproductive health. I wish I could make every person who has ever made a woman feel inferior because of her body or her desires or her shame or her grief read this essential anthology."
—Michele Filgate, editor of *What My Mother and I Don't Talk About* and *What My Father and I Don't Talk About*

"A beautiful and profoundly relatable collection of personal stories rooted in women's bodily and health care experiences. These essays will resonate with any woman who has been amused, horrified, confused, or delighted by our wild, bloody bodies. The juxtaposition of a public simultaneously obsessed with and profoundly negligent toward women's bodies and reproduction is laid bare with humor and heartbreak. What a wonderful collection!"
—Christine Murphy, author of *Notes on Surviving the Fire*

"In true feminist tradition, *So Heavy a Weight* shows us that the personal and the political are inseparable. Between the covers lies a choir of voices narrating, loudly and clearly, that which we have been taught is un-sayable, unspeakable, unseemly. This book is not only beautiful; it is necessary."
—Alekszandra Rokvity, PhD

"*So Heavy a Weight* journeys us through the lyrical, resilient, predictable and unpredictable joys, and challenges of the female body's reproductive life in its so many iterations. As I read these excellent contributions, I was struck by the range as much as the singularity of the voices, from accounts of menstruation, fertility programs, menopause, and miscarriages to the choice of whether to terminate a pregnancy or the ability to give birth. The revelation is always a realization that a woman's body is her own to inhabit and narrate. The obstacles to that realization are the imposed and socially mandated scripts these essays, individually and as a collection, deconstruct as they celebrate agency and the power to claim it."
—Adrianne Kalfopoulou, author of *Ruin: Essays in Exilic Living*;
On the Gaze: Dubai and Its New Cosmopolitanisms;
and *A History of Too Much*

"Muriel Rukeyser wrote that 'if one woman told the truth about her life . . . the world would split open.' Imagine, then, what happens when twenty-seven women tell their truths. By collecting these widely varied, heartfelt stories of pain, wit, and resilience, writer/editor Stephanie Vessely reminds us that personal experience is political—and that no one carries the weight alone."
—Chip Livingston, author of *Museum of False Starts*
and *Crow-Blue, Crow-Black*

"*So Heavy a Weight* offers up a collection of essays that speak to the shared experience of AFAB folx navigating a society that seems designed to work against us. These poignant essays touch on the familiar themes of menstruation, menopause, abortion, miscarriage, and everything in between, delivering relatable storytelling that acknowledges the lack of discussion and education around the inner workings of our bodies, while simultaneously challenging the stigma surrounding these topics."
—Victoria Patt-Timmerman,
Certified Health Education Specialist

"Some anthologies are poised at the right moment but don't seem particularly intense in their explorations of subject. Others contain work that might be individually electric but lack the thematic cogency a collection requires. *So Heavy a Weight*, under Stephanie Vessely's acute editorship, manages to accomplish both of these difficult goals. It is a timely subject, fiercely so, approached by wildly talented writers such as Marcia Aldrich, Jill Talbot, Sonya Huber, Abigail Thomas, Aileen Weintraub, the editor herself, and others, equally accomplished. The range of forms, from short lyrical essay to imagined interview, prose dialogue to list, is impressive, but most important is the range and depth of women's reproductive experiences represented in this stirring, sometimes wrenching, and necessary anthology."

—David Lazar, co-editor of *20th Century Essays*, Ohio State University Press

"A must-read for every woman, yes, but also, believe it or not, for any man. I had to put this book down every so often to collect myself. Some of the essays rattled me; others stirred feelings of guilt and shame for my lifelong neglect or willful ignorance of women's stories. But mostly, I empathized, sensing the longing behind every essay—for understanding, for self-acceptance, for voice."

—David Hicks, author of *The Gospel According to Danny*

So Heavy a Weight

Creative Writers on Women's Reproductive Health

Edited by Stephanie Vessely

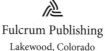

Fulcrum Publishing
Lakewood, Colorado

Copyright © 2025 Stephanie Vessely

All rights reserved. No part of this book may be reproduced or transmitted in any form or by any means, electronic or mechanical, including photocopying, recording, or by any information storage and retrieval system, without permission in writing from the publisher.

Library of Congress Cataloging-in-Publication Data
On file at the Library of Congress

Cover design by Kateri Kramer

Printed in the United States of America
0 9 8 7 6 5 4 3 2 1

Fulcrum Publishing
7333 W. Jefferson Ave., Suite 225
Lakewood, CO 80235
(800) 992-2908 • (303) 277-1623
www.fulcrumbooks.com

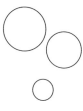

Contents

Introduction | xi
  Stephanie Vessely

Post | 1
  Emma Bolden

By the Numbers | 7
  Melissa Anderson

These Rooms Alone: A Conversation | 13
  Jill Talbot and Marcia Aldrich

Fog Warning | 21
  Julie Hohulin

Secrets | 25
  Sari Fordham

Notes for the Babysitter | 31
  Lori Sebastianutti

Old Birds and Empty Nests | 35
  Sonya Huber

The Antidote | 39
  Abigail Thomas

Becoming Your Own Sexual Advocate: A History of Oppression and the Victories Involving Reproductive Rights | 41
  Hillary Leftwich

losslist™ | 51
  Sarah Swandell

An Imagined Conversation with My Local School District in Which I Advocate for Heavily Menstruating Students | 57
  Joy Victory

Barren: A Journey | 63
 Alyse Knorr

Hold On, It's a Rough Ride | 71
 Angelique Fawns

Seeds | 77
 Yoda Olinyk

Anonymous Question Box for Eve | 83
 Deborah Meltvedt

Blood Rites | 91
 Katey Funderburgh

One | 99
 Katie Clausen

A Story of Two Births | 109
 Jennifer Alessi

Into the Dark | 115
 Stephanie Vessely

Self-Defense Posture | 123
 Monica Prince

A Weight Too Heavy | 135
 Leah Mueller

On Being So-Called Sensitive | 141
 Chloe Caldwell

Monsters: An Excerpt from *Knocked Down:
A High-Risk Memoir* | 147
 Aileen Weintraub

Such a Big Word | 155
 Arielle Dance

The Five Stages of Out-of-Place Grief | 161
 Sammi LaBue

Back at Day One Again | 167
 Abby Koenig

Source Acknowledgments | *175*
Author Biographies | *177*

We are volcanoes.
When women offer our experience as our truth,
as human truth, all the maps change.
There are new mountains.

—Ursula K. Le Guin

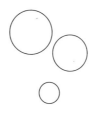

Introduction

I was twenty-nine when I had my first abortion. I was in a kind of/sort of relationship with the father at the time. We had been dating on and off for a year and half. He hadn't wanted to be in a relationship. He was divorced, with two children he was estranged from. It's more complicated than that, but the gist of the story is that we weren't on any kind of track toward marriage or building a family someday, no matter how badly I would have liked that to be true. He was clear from the beginning: He did not ever want to get married again. He did not want any more children.

I got pregnant because I timed my menstrual cycle wrong. I had stopped taking birth control pills because my boyfriend and I were technically broken up, and because the pills made me moody and depressed and crazy. I thought I was in the safe part of my cycle—the part when my ovaries have not yet released an egg and therefore it cannot be fertilized—so I didn't push my partner to wear a condom. This fact sticks with me—at twenty-nine, I didn't know the very basic biological fact that sperm can live inside the body for days after ejaculation. When I ovulated a day or two later, it was the perfect timing for sperm and egg to meet.

My boyfriend/not-boyfriend knew I was pregnant before I did. I was in denial. My period had been late plenty of times. I had had pregnancy scares. But my period always arrived, usually when I stopped worrying about it—i.e., after I took a test that confirmed I wasn't pregnant. For a week I diligently checked my underwear every time I went to the restroom. I had phantom cramps. I kept thinking my period would come. That it had to come. I attributed my breast soreness to PMS. The tightness of my pants to bloating. It took me a week to buy a test, because I think some part of me knew.

I still have a hard time describing the moment I saw the word "pregnant" through the little window of the test. How it felt. The gut punch of it. The terror of it. The sadness of it. The loneliness of it. That feeling is locked inside my body forever. I immediately fell to my knees on my bathroom rug and began to cry. It sounds dramatic, but it's the truth.

The other truth is that I struggled for years after my abortions (I had another one the following year—same complicated boyfriend, same mistake, because it would be years until I learned the fact about sperm inside the body). I didn't have anyone to talk to about the abortions. I didn't even think I was allowed to talk about them. I looked everywhere for other women's stories but only found stories pushed by Christians in disguise—women who regretted their abortions and had found their way back to God. Instead of working through my feelings, I stuffed every single one—shame, anger, grief, gratitude, and more—deep inside and tried to carry on as if none of it had happened. Which, as anyone who has ever had to carry a secret or pretend for a long period of time knows, didn't lead anywhere good. My life got harder. Messier. I drank. A lot. I developed an eating disorder. I lost friends and distanced myself from family.

Eventually, I started putting pen to page. In doing so, I found a place to put everything I was feeling—a place that wasn't inside my body. And as I began to tell my story and share my writing, other women began to respond. I didn't know I knew so many people who had also had abortions. They were all around me. All that time I was grieving and alone and afraid, there were people right there I could have talked to. But because our culture is what it is, I didn't know. In sharing I found a kind of healing. And if not a resolution, at least a kind of peace.

Which is all to say that I believe in the power of words—to educate, to connect, to heal, to grow, to share, to lighten the load. That is one reason why I wanted to put this anthology together. Because the more we tell our stories, the better off we all are—we become more connected, less afraid. We become more knowledgeable and, hopefully, more empathetic.

I also wanted to edit this collection because of what I wrote earlier about being a full-grown woman who didn't know the basic biology of her body. How, I want to know, was I never taught such basic facts about ovulation? (The circumstances of my pregnancies were a mystery to me until at least a decade later, when I stumbled across a random sentence in a random article.) How do women not know they have fibroids or endometriosis— or how to treat them? How do we still struggle with infertility, menopause, pregnancy, miscarriage, menstruation? How do we not have more answers by now, more direction? How are we still so in the dark when it comes to how our bodies work and what we are carrying with us every day?

This isn't a collection that purports to have the answers (although I'm fairly certain the answers lie in the fact that most medical research to date has been done on men's bodies[1]). This is not a medical book or any kind of guide. Rather, it is meant to shed light onto what it's like to be a woman today. To give voice to the myriad stories—heartbreaks, triumphs, pains, struggles, uncertainties—women carry with them every day. But it's not meant to be all-encompassing. It can't be. In selecting the essays for this anthology, I read through hundreds of stories about everything from medical mishaps to outright medical negligence. There were stories of devastating losses, infuriating injustices. There was questioning, confusion, longing. There was joy too. And humor. The pages that follow are only a small sample of the stories that are out there. It's impossible to cover women's reproductive health to the extent it deserves. It's impossible to cover every topic, period.

I would be remiss if I didn't also mention the *Dobbs v. Jackson Women's Health Organization* decision as also being a motivator behind this collection. In the days after the ruling, I told friends that I legitimately felt like less of a person. I was full of a kind of rage that scared me a little bit—a rage that only intensified when I saw tweets celebrating the loss of our freedoms. All I could think about was how many men have benefited from abortion—the countless lives made possible by our choices. I thought about my former partner, his current life, and how it exists because of what I went through. I wondered how many of those celebrating senators and judges and congressmen have secret abortions hiding in their closets. How many men wouldn't be where they are today if they had had that baby in high school or college? If their mistress had had that baby? Would they be less willing to take away our rights if they had to face the consequences of what they did?

But I digress.

If I learned anything from the experience of putting this book together, it's how much women hold at all times. I've witnessed the struggles of my friends and family—early or daunting menopause, fertility issues, painful periods, unexplained maladies—and I've had my own experiences. But it's easy to forget it all, to look past it in the busyness of our lives. There's something about reading story after story back-to-back that gets ahold of you. That reminds you that every single one of us is dealing with something. Carrying something. Holding something. We are grieving or we are in pain. We are hopeful or we are disappointed. We are tired, questioning, confused, lost. And we are all these things while raising kids and grandkids, while going to school, while working full time, while dealing with chronic pain and other ailments, while struggling financially or worrying that the money is going to run out someday. It's so much. I don't know how we hold it all. But we do.

I hope that these essays will help us lighten the load a little bit and remind us, as clichéd and trite as it might sound, that we aren't alone.

Reference

1. Gabrielle Jackson, "The Female Problem: How Male Bias in Medical Trials Ruined Women's Health," *The Guardian* (November 13, 2019), https://www.theguardian.com/lifeandstyle/2019/nov/13/the-female-problem-male-bias-in-medical-trials.

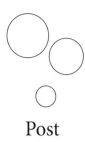

Post

Emma Bolden

Here is the thing you need to know first.

At the age of thirty-three, as a single woman who had no children, I underwent a total hysterectomy, meaning the removal of my uterus, ovaries, and fallopian tubes. By this point I had struggled for over twenty years with endometriosis, fibroid tumors, polycystic ovarian syndrome (PCOS), and extremely heavy and painful periods that sometimes lasted for six months. According to my medical history, the hysterectomy may have seemed like a choice. According to my actual life, it was a necessary step for me to be able to continue to live and work independently.

In other words, my story—my life and the choices I made within it—was controlled in ways that could accurately be described as "completely" by forces within my body I could not control.

When I started my period, I thought everyone would know. Instantly and just by looking at me. Everyone—I was sure of it—would *know*. This was, perhaps, understandable: I was just a kid, ten years old, and it made no sense to me that so great and fundamental a change could be a secret, hidden inside of my body and away from everyone who passed. It is perhaps not so understandable that I felt the same way when I had my hysterectomy. Everyone would know. I was certain. And so it was difficult for me to walk around in the world. It was difficult to look even a stranger in the eye. I didn't want to see myself there. I didn't want to see reflected the person I had no choice but to become.

***

Of course, when I had my hysterectomy, nobody knew. I didn't talk about it. I didn't even tell family members beyond my parents.

Like an action in any story, this had its consequences.

Not long after my hysterectomy, I traveled to a university for a conference. I served on a panel with a woman I online-knew and respected deeply. An audience member asked about daily writing routines. I began to describe mine. By "daily writing routine," I did not mean "the processes I have developed to stay somewhat sane." I meant "the only thing that, for a few moments, gives my mind something to focus on besides the amount of pain I am still in, which is a great deal, and how out of control I feel, which is an even greater deal."

After a hysterectomy, a person's abdominal organs shift to fill the absence, the space of what once existed. This shift can cause damage: a weakened pelvic floor, incontinence. The patient may be able to avoid the damage with physical therapy—Kegel exercises and breathing exercises and aerobics. Maybe. Sometimes, there is nothing one can do. A body does what it has to do to fill the absence, and the person inside that body has no choice but to deal with it.

The metaphor here is too easy, and so I'm not going to make it. Nothing is easy about this. Nothing.

As I talked about the importance of routine, of ritual, of doing something that feels like useful writing-related progress every day, the woman I deeply respect slid the microphone closer to her mouth.

"You can only do that because you didn't have children," she said. Childlessness was a privilege that allowed me time to write.

In second grade I rode my bike over a pothole, then hit the asphalt. Hard. So hard the breath left my body, and I sat there, trying and trying to breathe. And that's how I felt, after she spoke. Trying and trying. To breathe.

I tried to explain. I tried to say that no, I didn't have kids, that this was not exactly my choice, that I had in fact faced an impossible decision: have a hysterectomy or continue living with so much pain and bleeding that I was hardly living at all. Nothing I said mattered to her. I saw it in her eyes. And nothing I said mattered to me, either. I saw it in my own eyes in the bathroom mirror, where I rushed as soon as the panel was over.

My hormone replacement regimen still wasn't right—that would take four years, at least—and I was acutely aware of my body, of its sweat and stink, of how intensely I smelled of the three Starbucks lattes I'd downed after a sleepless night. I waited until I was alone in the bathroom to cry. I pulled my feet up so they wouldn't be visible from outside the stall. I wished I could just disappear. Vanish. I was acutely aware of how unfair the world was, how I was part of what made it unfair. I couldn't get over the guilt.

Because she was right. I felt like I had betrayed someone—her, myself, every parent who desperately wishes for a spare hour in a spare room with a spare notebook. The fact that I hadn't chosen not to be a parent made me no less guilty. In the wake of what she said, I couldn't see my achievements as anything other than luck, the result of a privilege I'd stubbornly insisted on calling a tragedy.

***

I wasn't angry at the woman on my panel. I couldn't be. After all, years earlier, I did the same thing.

Another conference. Another panel. A panelist talked about his own writing routine—and how, while he wrote, his wife cleaned and cared for the children, cooked and paid bills and performed all of the duties necessary to keep a house standing on its foundations. After he'd finished, I said that things were different when you were the one with the duties. I was imagining myself as the self I expected to be in ten years' time, in a house loud with children, bright with plastic bins of plastic toys. I hadn't yet imagined a life in which that wouldn't happen. In fact, I never imagined myself in the life I ended up having—not a mother, not even a cool aunt—at all.

Having children had been part of my narrative, albeit a ghostly one, since I was thirteen, when a doctor first told me it'd be difficult for me to get pregnant, that I'd need to try earlier rather than later. By *ghostly* I mean invisible yet present. I mean the invisible force behind every decision—the car I bought, the career I chose, the jobs I took. I always believed that I'd have children, and so surely that I built my life around that belief. When the possibility that I might have children was gone, the life remained and I had to keep living in it, like a character in a story that no longer belonged to her.

Now, it does not escape me that both of the incidents I describe took place at writers conferences. But it took me years to understand that the issue at hand is one of narrative, of the kinds of stories we tell about women and their wants and loves and lives. There's a difference between feeling like something is missing and feeling like something is missing because you're constantly being told it is, because stories like yours aren't part of the cultural narrative. And when motherhood is centered as the primary role for women, admitting you're happy without it can feel like a taboo. A sin.

This is so dire, I think to myself as I'm writing. *So regressive. It can't be true.* And then I consider how nearly every narrative I've read about infertility ends with motherhood, whether through miracle or medicine or adoption. In nearly every narrative I've read about childlessness, the women are insane, bitter monsters confined to often-literal attics. I wonder if I'd see myself differently if I saw women like me on paper, on screen, whole and fulfilled and happy. I wonder what it would be like to read or see stories where motherhood isn't part of the conflict or the resolution.

It isn't that I think we should have fewer stories about motherhood. Far from it. These narratives are absolutely essential, and we need more of them. More of the triumphs and tragedies, the daily and nightly bliss and sorrow and terror of the experience. More of every shade of doubt and despair and frustration, every quiet flush of happiness, every heart-flooding joy. We need narratives from every perspective: people of color, nontraditional families, queer families, trans and nonbinary parents. What I *am* saying is that not everyone can have children. Not everyone wants to have children. And if the only kind of narrative we tend to see—particularly about people who struggle with fertility or with diseases like endometriosis, fibroids, and PCOS—puts having children at the center of every conflict with some form of parenthood as the only resolution, it makes it difficult for people who can't or don't want to have children to see themselves. It makes it difficult, too, for other people to see them, in the sense of the word that implies understanding.

***

I didn't know how to talk about my hysterectomy. I didn't think I *could* talk about my hysterectomy, period, just like I didn't think I could talk about periods. It felt forbidden. A taboo. The kind of thing not to be discussed. It was so heavy a weight. I didn't want to say the words that would force someone, for the duration of the conversation, to take the responsibility of holding that weight with me. Or knowing it about me, having it there like a boulder at the back of the mind every time they thought of me.

I'm not sure why I thought in these terms other than that I had no way of thinking in other terms. It's what my hysterectomy was for me, after all: a giant, heavy boulder that shadowed every moment before and after it happened. And it wasn't even that I regretted it. I had done the thing that freed me, at least somewhat, from the cage of my own body. It also made me different from my peers in an entirely new way. My possibilities didn't match up with those of my friends, who were starting to get serious and get married, who were thinking about getting pregnant. It felt like a burden, this difference, and so I decided without even deciding that it was one better carried in silence, by which I mean alone.

You may wonder if I'm glad that I had a hysterectomy. It's a question I have asked myself many times, and every time, the answer is an automatic yes. But I don't fully know what's behind that yes. I don't know if that yes exists because I am glad to be rid of it—the blood and the blood, the moods that swung with wrecking-ball abandon through my teens and twenties. I don't know if instead I am glad to be rid of the questions I could never seem to run or talk or sleep away from: Would I be able to have my own children? Could I beat my body's clock, or would my body's clock stop on me? How would my story be resolved?

Now I know. There's a difference between a resolution and an ending. One is nothing like the other, but with both, there's a peace that comes afterward. A ceasing of tension, of conflict. Of possibility. There's a part of a story that's over enough to let you just be.

There is something to be said for just having an ending. There is something to be said for just letting yourself, whoever and however you are, be.

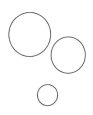

By the Numbers

Melissa Anderson

15—age at which my cousin got pregnant and I, five years old, did not understand how it was possible because my limited awareness of how babies arrived was that grownups who loved each other very much kissed and promised to have a baby together. I don't know how I came to this assumption, but it would be several years before someone corrected it.

10—age at which I got my first period at the end of fifth grade. I cried, ashamed and embarrassed that my body had betrayed me by maturing too early, not in junior high or high school like all the health classes had led me to believe.

15—age at which a boy kissed me for the first time outside my house after dark, and my mom opened the door and told me to get inside, and then yelled at me that she didn't want me making out with some boy in the parking lot like the girl next door.

18—age when I met a sophomore boy during freshman year of college who became my first real boyfriend.

8-12—number of condoms taped to the RA's door in the dorm, accessible all hours of the day and night, discreetly, without having to ask.

15—times my boyfriend begged to skip the condom he pulled off the door.

1—times I gave in to his pleas and made him promise to stop in time.

2—number of morning-after pills when I panicked after that one time, taken while sitting on the curb outside the campus health clinic. My boyfriend speculated about how a baby with our mix of DNA might look: a girl with dark, curly ringlets and dark eyes, his button nose, my smile. Part Hispanic, part white, part Black, with my intelligence and, perhaps, his sadness. My boyfriend said if I didn't want to take the Pill and if I did end up pregnant, he would drop out of school to support us. But even then, I knew he was not the one.

4—number of classes said boyfriend failed at the end of the second semester we were together, for which he blamed me; also, number of months until he broke up with me after I took those pills.

4,838—number of birth control pills taken over the course of a lifetime.

6—number of times my best friend lectured me over Instant Messenger about the evils of birth control and its poisonous chemicals while touting the rhythm method.

7:02—a.m., time when said best friend texted me that she needed to talk. When I called her on a break from work, she told me she was pregnant, maybe six weeks, and she couldn't *be* pregnant.

277—miles away she lived when I offered to go with her to a clinic. She said she didn't need me; she had a friend who would go. I never knew if it was the man who had impregnated her or someone else who drove her.

1—number of times in graduate school a male professor warned me not to have sex in South Africa because of HIV/AIDS before I left for a summer internship there. He did not give that same warning to the men in my class.

25—age at which my ob-gyn told me to start taking folic acid "just in case" even though I was single at the time with no intention of getting pregnant.

50—the percentage of pregnancies my ob-gyn said were unplanned, even among married couples.

435—dollars, the cost of a full STD panel *with* my company health insurance after a fling with a guy who said he was clean, but whom I later discovered had a girlfriend when we'd hooked up so I couldn't really trust him.

0—number of positive results from said panel.

400—dollars, amount my sister and I loaned to a cousin for an abortion when she got pregnant at thirty-eight just after losing a job and breaking up with a guy. She never paid us back.

30—age at which my biological clock kicked into high gear, and I desperately wanted a baby.

35—age by which I vowed to adopt a baby alone if I were still single.

2—blind dates I agreed to go on the year I turned thirty because of aforementioned clock.

31—age at which I connected to an old crush on Facebook.

32—age at which said crush DM'ed me and we made plans to hang out.

2—number of dates before I told crush that I wasn't interested in a fling because I needed to have a baby by the age of thirty-five.

60—second pause before crush responded back that he was also looking for something serious.

4—months before crush said he loved me.

II—cervical dysplasia level diagnosed by a colposcopy after an abnormal Pap smear result, followed by a biopsy, followed by a loop electrosurgical excision procedure (which sounds as awful as it is).

6—months before follow-up Pap smear determined all dysplasia was gone and months of extreme fear over my health, future fertility, and cost of treatment subsided.

3—doses of HPV vaccine that could have prevented it all if it had been available when I was a teen.

14—months of dating before crush proposed.

15—months of engagement before our wedding date.

4—average number of children families had who were featured in a rhythm method video we had to watch to get married in the Catholic church.

-3—months before the wedding when aunts pressured me to go off the pill and start trying to get pregnant because I wasn't getting any younger and I wouldn't be showing at the wedding if I was still early in the pregnancy. I did not oblige.

6—pregnancy tests in the first half year of marriage as we tried to get pregnant.

1—diagnosis of chronic illness with the recommendation to go back on the pill before getting pregnant.

16—nights in Ireland to stave off disappointment about putting off a pregnancy.

32—age at which an acquaintance who worked as a human rights advocate, a fellow University of Southern California grad (a lawyer in the making, who campaigned for President Obama), was diagnosed with stage IV cervical cancer. She did not survive the year.

1—onesie purchased for my sister's baby-to-be upon her receiving a positive pregnancy test.

4—nights my sister spent in the hospital due to an ectopic pregnancy after the medicine given to end the pregnancy failed and she ended up with a burst fallopian tube that required emergency surgery.

0—times my sister tried to get pregnant again.

4—number of family members and close friends who suffered miscarriages and stillbirths while my husband and I waited for the green light to try to get pregnant.

1—appointment with a perinatologist to discuss getting pregnant at a geriatric age with preexisting conditions.

5—dollars, cost of perinatology appointment with new, better employer health insurance.

5—ovulation test kits purchased when my husband and I decided we were ready to try again.

3—months of trying with negative pregnancy tests.

3—number of times I cried.

2—sunflowers a coworker left on my desk after the last negative test.

1—trip to Germany for a summer conference, during which I purchased a tiny wooden cradle Christmas tree ornament as a good luck charm.

1—lunch with my husband in which we discussed the limits to which we were willing to go to have a child. No IUI, no IVF, no adoption.

6—months we gave ourselves to try to get pregnant before we agreed to accept it wasn't in the cards for us.

98.9—basal body temperature on the first day I started tracking.

5—number of wineries visited for my sister-in-law's bachelorette party at which I offered to be the designated driver because we were in the waiting window to test again.

19—number of times I had to pee that day.

7:30—p.m., time I went to bed at a hotel in Lodi because I was exhausted.

4—days I waited to take a pregnancy test after the trip.

2—minutes it took for the pregnancy test to register a positive result.

38—age at conception.

2–3—weeks the digital pregnancy test estimated for how far along I was.

6—stress tests to monitor baby's heart rate in the last weeks of pregnancy.

4—methods of induction used: misoprostol, Pitocin, a Foley balloon, and manual breaking of the water.

58—hours of labor in the hospital from induction to a resident suggesting a C-section.

5—cm dilated at which labor stopped progressing.

20—minutes, length of C-section surgery.

5—number of days in the hospital after delivery due to baby's jaundice and my elevated blood pressure.

10—bonus days with baby before due date.

0—cost of eight days in the hospital, C-section delivery, and treatment of baby in bili lights crib with exceptional employer health insurance.

39—age at which an ob-gyn first recommended an IUD, after I had my first child, allowing me to stop thinking about birth control daily.

>—the opportunities I had to get an education and build a career by having a child on my own timeline with the partner of my choice.

∞—the cost to my niece, who is six months old, because she has been born into a world where conservative politicians and judges, who have all the power and privilege, will do everything they can to erode women's rights.

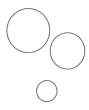

These Rooms Alone: A Conversation

Jill Talbot and Marcia Aldrich

I knew I was pregnant the moment my boyfriend fell back onto his side of the bed. I pulled the blue blanket over my naked body, willing it not to be so.

In elementary school, when we were bored in social studies or math, we'd play MASH, but only the girls. We'd write the letters for mansion, apartment, shack, and house at the top; 1, 2, 3, and 4 (for number of children) on the bottom; the names of four boys (for the men we might marry) on the left; and four types of vehicles on the right. Then we'd draw a spiral in the center, count the lines, and begin moving around the square. Our future in pencil. I don't remember enjoying the game or trusting in it the way the other girls in fifth grade did, their hushed giggles. Most girls didn't like it when I added a 0 to the children, RV to the housing, a category of careers instead of men. That's not how you're supposed to play.

We were raised to follow the narrative of life—college, marriage, career, children—as if this were the only story. In my twenties, I started checking off items like I was playing MASH. I didn't get far. During my first semester of graduate school, I listened to a nurse on the phone tell me I was pregnant, and when

I told my boyfriend of four years, he proposed. This is an odd detail, but that afternoon he had bought a new watch. I remember staring at the black band and feeling the spiral tighten, my choices being crossed out. I said no to all of it. This was not the story I wanted.

***

It took me a long time to realize I was pregnant, to realize I was carrying something inside me.

Unlike most of my girlfriends in high school, I had never dreamed about a future filled with children. I did not make lists of possible names for those children or talk about whether I wanted girls or boys. My friends knew they wanted two boys and two girls and what they would name them. Not for a single second did I look ahead and see myself with a child. Was there something wrong with me, something missing—did I lack the maternal gene? I felt I was supposed to want children and look forward to that day when they would arrive. It was the culmination of my two older sisters' desires when they became mothers. It was assumed I shared their desires, but I did not. In my fantasies I had multiple lovers but remained unattached to any. I was a singer, an actress, and finally a writer: my essential solitude the common thread. Never was there a child waiting in the wings for me to hold.

***

After reading your words, I went on a walk to think about what it was I wanted in high school. I went back to my mind at sixteen, at seventeen, those years when decisions were made for me, when I didn't think beyond the borders of Texas because no one else did, and my parents never offered it as an option, having never left the state themselves. I didn't grow up in a small town, but it felt that way. On my walk, I remembered, clearly, how I had hoped for one thing—to be far away. The rest of my yearnings I don't remember, not really.

I've always felt the pull of elsewhere, somewhere I don't yet see. How that desire perplexed me at a young age because I couldn't name it, just fought against all those who tried to warn me against myself. And there were many. *You think you want this now, but you'll see.* By the time I finished college, most of the people I knew were still living in my hometown or returning to it, having children, buying houses, choosing color schemes. I respected their lives, I did, but I didn't see that for myself. What I wanted was still far away, and it wasn't until graduate school—when I sat in professors' offices listening to them tell me I must keep going, I must pursue a PhD—that I recognized my secret self, ambition. Everything I wanted, I wanted alone.

***

I don't know exactly when I got pregnant. I can't say what I might have felt at the time of conception except to say the last thing on my mind was making a baby. It was not a momentous occasion. I've read about sex being enhanced because the couple thought they might be making a baby—that thought never touched me. It only finally occurred to me I might be pregnant because my symptoms couldn't be explained by anything else. You see, the father had been told after undergoing tests that he was sterile. Until those tests, I had dutifully used a diaphragm, carrying it around with me in its blue plastic case with the accompanying tube of spermicide. I hated the thing, but I used it because I knew the worst thing that could happen to me was to become pregnant. At nineteen, I had nothing about me to recommend I become a parent. About a great many things, I was unsure; about my unsuitability to be a mother, I was certain.

***

My boyfriend and I met in college and dated, off and on, for a total of four years. He followed me to graduate school, to Lubbock, where he got a job teaching history at one of the middle schools in town. I was twenty-three. I was following the narrative of life. Begrudgingly. Our relationship felt weary, obligatory at times, something I'd try to break free from every few months, but here we were, together. Here we were, under a gray sky bearing down without the deluge. And here we were, driving to a nondescript building one morning in October, the day after I sat through a counseling session with a nurse, who told me about my body and what it carried in an office that looked like a craft area for a kindergarten class. I restated my choice, my decision, my certainty; then I listened to the steps of the procedure, how long I would bleed, when to call a doctor. Did I understand? Was I sure? If so, come back in the morning at seven. Don't eat anything after midnight. We'll give you a Valium. I remember my only worry: how we would pay for it. The next morning, I wasn't surprised by the gathered protestors outside the Women's Clinic on 67th in their coats of indignation, their posters of blood and Bible verses. I was surprised by the crowded waiting room, all ages and races, the way we tried to give one another the privacy we had surrendered in the parking lot. I slumped down into the Valium, considered the affluent couple in the corner, their gray hair and look of shock, as if their bodies had betrayed them. I remember the numbing shot in my cervix and a painting of blue flowers on the wall and the sound of the vacuum and the way I trembled in the recovery room, sipping Sprite from a plastic cup and throwing up into a trash can and being told it was time to leave.

***

When the father was pronounced sterile, the outcome did not surprise him, though it surprised me. I had never considered not being able to get pregnant, since I lived in constant fear that I would get pregnant. According to the doctor, there was some minuscule possibility I could conceive. The word "miracle" was used. I remember that. After receiving the doctor's prognosis, I stopped using birth control, secure in the medical knowledge I couldn't get pregnant. In late September, I was beset by all manner of physical symptoms I couldn't explain. Without telling Bruce, I went to the health clinic on campus, where I described what turned out to be morning sickness and was told I must be pregnant. I protested but took the test, and sure enough, six months after the doctor's declaration of Bruce's sterility, I was pregnant.

I did not run home to share the good news with Bruce. I called it a mistake, the latest in a long line of terrible mistakes I had been making or that had befallen me since I had met Bruce. It never occurred to me that this might be the only child he might conceive, his one chance at parenthood. Picture a young woman, more like a teenager, who finds herself pregnant, and all she can feel is a desperate fear. Perhaps she isn't a sympathetic character; perhaps she should have felt maternal stirrings, but she did not. There was nothing but the sense that with each passing day, she was losing more of who she was, and she had already lost too much.

***

It was the years after, for me, when I lost myself—in drinking, in danger—but it wasn't the aftershock from that October morning. I am sure of that, though the years with Dean had something to do with what became a recklessness in me. When I left Lubbock to pursue my PhD, I learned to act as if there were no rules except the ones I ignored.

Dean and I get back to his apartment, and I crawl into bed drowsy and queasy. I pull the blue blanket over me while he paces the hallway, his athletic figure darting back and forth in the door frame. The air conditioner clicks on, because this is Texas, and twenty years from now, in 2013, the House will close the clinic we just left, along with half of the others in the state. I begin to doze off, hear the jingle of keys, and call after him, a question. "You have to stay with me, in case I hemorrhage," I say, but he looks toward the front door and mumbles, "Call the school." I hear the key turn in the lock and shuffle to the bathroom. Make sure. What I did, I understand, I did alone. I want to be kind, to say Dean couldn't handle what he had seen that morning, but he saw only a waiting room and fists pounding on his truck when we pulled out of the parking lot. We stayed together out of some perverse, young-person view that if we had gone through such a thing together, we had to honor it. When he proposed again that next spring, I said yes. Surely there's a word other than mistake.

***

In 1970 the state of New York led the way, offering legal abortion on demand through the twenty-fourth week of pregnancy. The US Supreme Court's landmark decision in *Roe v. Wade* wouldn't legalize abortion nationwide until 1973. Unlike one of my high school friends who had to fly to Mexico for an abortion and another who was secretly admitted to a high-end clinic, I made an appointment over the phone with Planned Parenthood.

It was a cold day when we drove to Syracuse. The day was gray, the waves choppy with small whitecaps, foamy, spraying when they rolled to the shore of Lake Cayuga, the wind biting. There was nothing fresh about the day.

We left early in the morning to make my appointment. The drive was silent. The decision had been made. There was nothing further to be said, and we didn't say the nothing that was. We parked in a lot by the nondescript building. I checked in at a small metal desk, filled out forms, verified I was eighteen, then was taken back to the medical part of the clinic. Bruce stayed in the waiting room, empty or nearly so, except for him.

I was treated kindly. I had a vacuum aspiration, and I remember the noise of the suction and the pain of the contractions. Then

I was moved to an empty recovery room and lay on a narrow bed. It was as if the clinic had been invented and staffed just for me.

***

My recovery room was a row of chairs against a wall in a very small room, more like a hallway. All I remember is white. Maybe it was the white gowns or the white trash can or the white cup I trembled in my hand. We were lined up, not looking at one another, huddled into ourselves until a nurse asked if we could stand. I wonder about the difference between the solitude of your narrow bed in the 1970s and a chair among many in a hallway twenty years later, but nothing's that different, not really, not even now, because we still shoulder these rooms alone. I told only one person back then—a long-distance phone call—a friend who responded by naming girls who snuck away for abortions before we even graduated high school.

One month before the wedding, Dean called to ask, "PhD or me?" I flew from Dallas, where my mother had bought me a white dress, and I sat in the Lubbock airport bar sipping wine when Dean walked in, resignation on his face. I understood—I could chase ambition or I could stay in Texas. I had to cross one of them out. I left Dean in the parking lot, then wandered the empty corridor of the airport in a daze until morning. I got on a plane, and I got on with my life. Later I would come to understand how I sidestepped a story I didn't want to live. Now, it's a story I tell.

***

I didn't tell anyone about the pregnancy and the abortion. It wasn't the sort of thing I'd share back then, and I had no one to share it with. Did I feel any regret? The girl I was felt relieved. I felt spared from a great calamity. And I felt grateful above all else that abortion was legal, that Bruce could afford to pay for it, and that I had someone who shared my feelings going forward with the decision. I felt lucky my life could resume. I held on to the idea that my getting pregnant wasn't my fault and that I had been given incorrect assurances I couldn't conceive. It was Bruce who felt guilty about what he put me through because, unbeknownst to him, he had passed along the doctor's false assessment and I got pregnant, I bore the consequences, I had to make the decision, and I had to undergo the procedure. It was me, not him, who would have to say I had an abortion when I was nineteen. He wouldn't have to admit a thing. I would have to reveal this piece of information for the rest of my life on medical forms. I would have to count myself among the countless women who had abortions. I would not stand apart, unscathed.

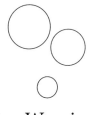

Fog Warning

Julie Hohulin

My eyes flutter open, and I find myself in that space between dreaming and fuming that I'm awake again. Less than an hour has passed since my last battle with consciousness. My pulse is racing, and a warmth is beginning to radiate from my core toward the surface of my now-clammy skin. There's a trickle of sweat between my boobs, in the bend of my elbows, and along my hairline. I try to focus on taking long, deep breaths, in and out, in and out. Somewhere I read that slowing your pulse during a hot flash will douse the blaze more quickly. It feels like a fire has been kindled in my core, and it's slowly consuming me from the inside out. My husband snores quietly beside me, oblivious to the combustion taking place on my side of the bed.

Then, as quickly as it starts, it's gone. And now I'm untangling the linen duvet I kicked off during the inferno and pulling it back up to my chin because I'm freezing. This sequence repeats itself two or three more times before a coveted morsel of oblivion is interrupted by my phone alarm telling me it's 6 a.m. Wake up, it's menopause.

A fun fact about night sweats—not only do they wreck any remnants of a good hair day, but they also prevent you from getting any real REM sleep at night. Which means I spend the daylight hours in a fog, forgetting why I picked up my phone or whether I wrote that thank-you note to my sister. Or worse, convincing my adult daughter that I'm not day drinking, just passing through that glorious passageway otherwise known as "the change of life."

Thankfully, my book club friends, all older than me, had warned me of the hot flashes, migraines, and insomnia that was to come. But no one mentioned that I might actually lose my mind. As a retired advertising executive, I thrived at juggling multiple deadlines and managing complex projects. Now, I can't load the dishwasher while making dinner without forgetting to add the chicken to the pot pie. I feel incompetent and even confused at times. Activities that used to be automatic somehow fall through the cracks, and I find myself apologizing for forgetting to pay the Nordstrom bill and neglecting to pick up olive oil, again.

What the fuck? At a time of life when I should be feeling accomplished and wise, I am second-guessing myself. I had anticipated physical changes as my body sheds its childbearing abilities, but I wasn't ready for the insecurity that comes from observing my once-sharp mind lose its edge to sleep deprivation and hormonal brain fog. A Google search of "menopause and mental clarity" reveals that my symptoms may last up to four years. Four years? It's highly possible I will burn down the condo before then!

Like any type A personality, I develop tricks for appearing in control. I make lists, leave myself Post-it Notes, and set alarms for everything—time to move the laundry, remember to preheat the oven, don't forget to sign up for yoga tomorrow. But in reality, there's one important reminder that I keep forgetting over and over again—the reminder that I am not alone.

Those of us who are lucky enough to have been born with the ability to produce eggs and those of us who are lucky enough to continue celebrating birthdays will likely experience some discomfort and confusion during menopause. It's natural, it's a part of life, and we don't need to be ashamed or afraid of it. In fact, we can demystify the transition by owning it, talking about it, sharing it with our sisters, our daughters, and the men in our lives. Especially with the men in our lives.

As I swing my legs out of bed, shove my feet into my worn slippers, and face another foggy day, I vow to give myself and others the support needed to pass through these years with grace and confidence. Repeat after me: "I am not crazy. I am not losing my mind. I am a wise and wonderful being evolving in body and spirit." Now, where did I put those coffee beans that I bought yesterday?

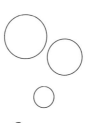

Secrets

Sari Fordham

The room is dark and hushed. I lie on the table and crane my neck to watch the screen. It looks like static. "Your bladder is full," the student tells me, gliding the transducer over my stomach. She is young enough to be my student, I think. I'm still wearing my teaching clothes, a buttoned-up shirt, my nicest jeans. My messenger bag, heavy with books and papers, slumps on a chair by the door.

I did not expect to be here, in this darkened room. At the obstetrician's office, I cheerfully answered questions—"Yes, I'm taking my vitamins. No, no morning sickness." At the end of the appointment, my obstetrician wheeled in a portable sonogram, gazed at the murky image, and sent me to this teaching hospital. "Try not to worry," she said as I left.

The student glides the transducer over my stomach, her eyes on the screen. "The real technician might come in," she tells me. "She might take over." Despite the student's discomfort or maybe because of it, I like her. I can tell she feels responsible for me.

She clicks to make an X. She clicks again, making another X. Then she measures the distance between the two. I'm curious how it all works. I have only seen sonograms on television, accompanied by reassuring swishing and a blurry fetus. What the student is doing looks more like someone's geometry homework.

"Do you see anything?" I ask. I feel intrusive, as if the content of my uterus is her secret.

"I'm not allowed to tell you," she says. "Your doctor will let you know."

"My doctor said I should only come back to her office if there's a problem. Otherwise, I can go home." The implication lingers.

"I'll ask the technician," she says.

My husband, Bryan, jokingly referred to me as the sacred vessel, knowing it would provoke. "How is the sacred vessel today?" he would say, all honey.

When we were roughhousing and I was losing, I would shout: "Sacred vessel! Sacred vessel!"

"It's going to be a long nine months," he said.

The student returns with the technician, who is young and blond and pregnant. I've always been appalled that strangers will reach toward a pregnant woman's stomach. Now I understand the impulse. I wonder how it feels to be so definitively with child. The technician looks at the marks the student has made. "Ovary," she says about one. "Fibroid," she says about another. She picks up the transducer and runs it over my stomach.

Come on, kid. Where are you?

I took two pregnancy tests. The first was a pale blue cross. The second, more assertive. "I think I'm pregnant," I said. I smiled. Bryan smiled. "Wow, we're really going to do this." The next day, the doctor confirmed it.

Still, we were cautious. I was cautious. We only told immediate family. When discussing the future, I would say awkwardly, "If we have a baby." A caveat.

"Twenty-five percent of pregnancies end in miscarriage," I told my sister breezily. An incorrect statistic, it turns out. The number is actually between 15 and 20 percent. In any case, I was no sentimental pregnant lady.

"We need a better image," the technician says. She directs me to the bathroom and tells me that after I've emptied my bladder, I should return, strip from the waist down, and wait. "You can cover with this," she says, handing me a white sheet.

Transvaginal ultrasounds have been in the news lately. State lawmakers, mostly men, are deciding whether or not they will force women to get one before an abortion. These laws will require doctors to describe the fetus, the heartbeat, information the woman is not requesting.

I have been watching the news angrily, hand over my stomach.

"Do you ever want kids?" Bryan asked me. We weren't dating yet. We were just two friends, canoeing and talking about life. I dipped my paddle into the lake and pulled on the handle, feeling the water's resistance.

I was a certified spinster. Thirty-four and never married. My sister Sonja was going through a divorce and considering what it meant to be single again. At her lawyer's office, she chatted with the receptionist about how I was single and happy. But no kids. Sonja had two sons. The receptionist had a daughter. They agreed that while a man was optional, children weren't. "Your sister needs to get pregnant before it's too late," the receptionist had advised.

I laughed when Sonja called to tell me. "Oh, goodness," I said. "I'm fine."

If I had children, would I even be canoeing? I taught in California, and in the summer, I was free to travel and to be on this Minnesota lake. The wind was kicking up the water, and we could hear loons calling in the distance. On the sandbar, mothers sat with their babies, taking pebbles from their hands, applying sunscreen. I didn't even own a pet because of the responsibility.

"Kids? I don't know," I told Bryan. "I'll see what happens."

I'm back quickly from the bathroom, and it doesn't take long to slide out of my jeans. I sit on the papery table as primly as I can without pants, without anything. I arrange and rearrange the sheet, and then I wait. My phone is in my messenger bag. I wonder if I have time to hop off the table, cross the room, and get it before they return. Bryan will be wondering about the appointment. I had called him from the hospital parking lot, anxious.

Do I text him? What would I even say?

A polite knock on the door, and the technician and the student return. The student picks up a probe. It is nearly two feet long and it looks like a plastic curling iron. "It doesn't go all the way in," she says helpfully.

After my sister's divorce, I drove to Tucson on all my school breaks. Sonja was raising her children alone *and* getting her PhD *and* teaching. She needed all the help she could get, and when I visited, she would leave before breakfast and return after the children were in bed. Aidan and Avery were five and two. In the mornings, they would jump on me and shout, "You're a T-Rex!"

We would hatch dinosaur eggs, make play-dough, build trains. It sounds like a lot more fun than it actually was. "Don't feel bad," Sonja would tell me late in the evening. "I get bored too. Kids can be boring."

When I visited, I would listen to children's music, change diapers, settle fights, put the offender in time-out, make lunch, wipe jam off faces, wrestle small bodies into and out of car seats, walk in the park, sing the same songs, read the same books. Only once did I have the nerve to go with them alone to the grocery store. We must have needed something vital like ketchup or coffee. By 3 p.m., I was exhausted. By their bedtime, I was catatonic.

How did Sonja do this day in and day out?

The next day, Aidan would be at my elbow: "Read me a book, mommy."

"I'm not your mommy," I would gently remind him.

The transvaginal ultrasound is intrusive. I have always been so modest. My mother used to tell me, "Good grief, you don't have anything special." Here on this table, I'm without shame. I'm interested only in the screen, the clicking, the silent communication between student and teacher. I am waiting for someone to say: *Don't worry. We can't tell you anything officially, but stress isn't good for the baby.*

The room is dark and hushed. Like church.

Over Christmas, Bryan and I drove to Tucson to visit my family. We had seven hours to choose a name.

"Sycamore," I said. "Rain," I said. "Here's a good one. What about Marilla?"

"I can't tell if you're joking or not," he said.

"Oh, I'm not."

"That's what I was afraid of."

We settled on a name for each gender. They were unusual enough for me, normal enough for him. We said them over and over as we passed chollas and saguaros. We agreed not to tell anyone. They were our secret.

I'm dressed, finally, and sitting on a chair. The ultrasound machine has been turned off, but the room is still dark. Outside, the technician and the student are discussing my uterus. I'm today's lesson, but what is it?

I pull out my phone and move my fingers across the buttons. I am careful to capitalize correctly.

I think I miscarried.

When my friends tell me I will only understand love when I become a mother, I want to roll my eyes. *A baby doesn't make a woman complete,* I want to say. *Your kids are cute, but you're a person too.* They mean well, these friends. They love their babies and cannot imagine being childless, and they're curious, I'm sure, how I would navigate my vocal feminism and motherhood. "Not every woman wants a baby," I say.

"A baby is not necessary," I later tell my sister, and I do believe it. I'm frustrated that there is only one acceptable life, that women who choose not to have children are looked at with pity. If they are young, they are told that they will change their minds, and if they are old, people will whisper—*Oh, it's too late for her now.* Men's self-worth is not linked as directly to procreation.

But here is my secret: I am not matter-of-fact. Despite my belief that babies don't make women complete, despite my tough talk, I have always wanted children. When I was a happy spinster, I would sometimes stand in the shower and think about babies, and my heart would tighten in panic. *I'm never having kids!* I would think. Then I would try to shake it off like a basketball injury. I would try to think about something else—papers I had to grade, lessons to plan.

The technician knocks. She crosses the room and faces me; her pregnant belly presses against the metal table between us. "You should go back and see your doctor," she says. "I've sent her the results."

As she pushes the box of tissues toward me, I vow to tell no one about this moment, about how lonely I feel, how hollowed out.

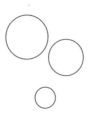

Notes for the Babysitter

Lori Sebastianutti

Hello to the *New Life Fertility Center* embryologist assigned to my file! Below are some important notes that will be helpful during the next five days while my embryos are under your care. I know that you've dedicated your life to helping people like me become parents, but after seven years and no baby, I thought I'd make sure we're on the same page! They're fairly detailed, but please don't hesitate to contact me if you have any questions.

Thanks!
Lori

Day 1

Please make sure the incubator is warm (37°C) and dark to best mimic the natural conditions of my fallopian tube. The fertilized eggs, or zygotes, must receive proper nourishment—a careful balance of carbon dioxide, oxygen, proteins, amino acids, and enzymes. Oh, and please don't forget to maintain the correct pH balance, as this is critical for their growth and survival!

If you need me, I'll be lying in bed, resting my grapefruit-sized ovaries. (Having multiple eggs removed from your follicles by way of a needle connected to a suction device is no walk in the park!)

I'll be watching a variety of reality television shows to keep my mind off the fact that my genetic offspring is growing in a lab. I'll also be trying not to think about the large sum of money that has just been charged to my credit card, nor all of the medications that are streaming through my body, like high-dose hormones, corticosteroids, and blood thinners.

P.S. Please tell my zygotes that I'm sorry I couldn't be there and that I really tried.

Day 2

Please remember not to disturb the zygotes today, as they need to grow from one cell to eight. This might be a good time for a few housekeeping items. Please ensure the following:
- All incubators are appropriately alarmed and monitored.
- An automatic emergency generator is ready in the event of a power failure.
- The filtered air within the lab is replaced several times per hour to prevent contaminants from interrupting the growth of embryos.
- A strict chain of custody protocol is in place to ensure the proper identification of samples at each stage of the process.

If you need me, I'll be at home, attempting to walk around, partaking in light activities, like making lunch or taking a shower. I won't be doing much, as everyone I know is at work or taking care of their children, and many of the friends I used to have are gone. I haven't been the easiest to deal with these last seven years.

P.S. Please tell my soon-to-be eight-cell embryos that I'm sorry I couldn't be there and that I really tried.

Day 3

Make sure to check on the embryos to see if they have reached eight cells (cleavage stage). If so, please ensure they are then moved into a new petri dish containing a culture that mimics the tissue fluids of the uterus, as this is the day they would travel to the uterine cavity in a spontaneous conception. Please confirm that this culture medium contains a higher level of sucrose because they'll need their energy to grow to approximately forty cells within the next twenty-four hours.

If you need me, I'll be at home inserting progesterone suppositories into my vagina. (I have to make my lining an ideal home for my embryos—plump and rich with blood!) I'll also be busy practicing what I learned during the last two years of counseling—repeating affirmations such as "Trust that all will unfold for the greatest good" and visualizing myself with a rounded belly or rocking a newborn baby in my arms. Every time I have a negative thought, I'll practice diaphragmatic breathing to ride out the anxiety that's hounded me since childhood.

P.S. Please tell my embryos that I'm sorry I couldn't be there and that I really tried.

Day 4

Today is another big growing day, so it's probably best to leave the embryos undisturbed. Compaction and early blastulation should occur as the embryos transform from a loosely associated group of cells to a more tightly compacted morula. They will also need their rest for transfer day tomorrow.

If you need me, I'll be kneeling in a church pew, praying that at least one of the embryos makes it to blastocyst. I will bargain with Jesus, Mary, and all the saints, promising middle names in their honor and years of unwavering devotion.

P.S. Please tell my morulae that I'm sorry I couldn't be there and that I really tried.

Day 5 (Homecoming Day!)

Please remove any viable blastocysts from the culture for their final assessment. If you see that at least one has three distinct layers—a fluid-filled cavity in the center; a flat layer of cells called the trophectoderm, which will become the placenta; and a clump of cells called the inner cell mass, which will become the baby—please load it in a soft catheter to be placed in my uterus by way of my cervix.

If you need me, I'll be heading to the clinic with an uncomfortably full bladder to ensure the doctor can view my reproductive organs on the ultrasound machine. I'll be holding my husband's free hand as he drives, thankful for his unfaltering support during these long, dark years, grateful that our marriage is still intact. I will be trying not to be overly hopeful that it decides to stick around for the next nine months, nonetheless thrilled that I get to reunite with it in its new form, even for just a short time.

P.S. Please tell my future child that I'm almost there.

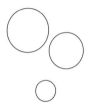

Old Birds and Empty Nests

Sonya Huber

I'm a little over six months into the empty nest experience. Friends warned me that the first month, in particular, might leave me weepy and overwhelmed. To be honest, I feel amazing. I look great because I've slept, and the stress of leaving my son at school has calmed down somewhat. And it's been a long time since I had impromptu sex in the kitchen.

Leaving him was one of those rites of passage that feel heavy and fiery because the moment has been so overwritten with the stories and images of others, and with my own memories. But I had practice, as I've been leaving him since he was four for visits with his father, who lives several states away. I've had to trust his well-being and his ability to navigate challenging situations, to fly and come back.

But that is the baby bird flying, not the nest. My son and I share a love of scavenging, picking up pieces of nature, so we've got nests and bones, skulls and feathers and rocks tucked into shelves and boxes. And a bird's nest is a marvel, each defined by a pattern associated with a species, created with local material, some messy and casual, some perfectly smooth inside like a teacup. The thing about a nest is that it's built to be empty. That's the nature of a cup, of any container: its emptiness, its holding capacity, is its strength.

The ability to craft a nest doesn't die when the baby bird leaves. The knowledge, the container-building developed and passed on from bird to bird, flies away with the bird who built it. The mother bird also leaves the nest, which disintegrates or which some lucky child finds on the ground as a message from the world that safety and care can be built from grass and mud.

I love the nest I grew my son in, the empty space of my uterus, but that is now also discarded. I was overjoyed to get rid of it in 2018, when I was forty-seven, because, like an old bird's nest, it got weird and crumbly. Fibroids bled and poked me whenever I had sex, and toward the end, I was buying stick-on pain patches and wearing them everywhere.

So I went into my gynecologist's office, and she did an ultrasound and said things didn't look too bad. She offered to check again in six months, but I'd seen enough of wait and see. I paused and said, "Y'know, if someone offered to give me a hysterectomy in the parking lot with a spoon, I'd take them up on it."

I still remember her widened eyes, the silent way she regarded me. To her credit, she listened and scheduled surgery. I expected to feel all the ways: less of a woman, closer to death, functionless—I don't know. I'm a crier, so I expected to feel sad and signed up for an online hysterectomy support group.

In the blur of recovery, my doctor came out of the operating room to show me pictures. "You were right," she said. "They were bigger than they looked on the ultrasound, and one was pressing right on your bladder with what looked like teeth!" They weren't teeth, but of course my uterus had grown its own kind of tissue-fangs.

I have to tell you: I love love love my uterine-free body. Within days, I felt AMAZING. I felt the way I remembered feeling as a preteen girl, rangy and blank in my belly, not weighted down with a squishiness that expanded and contracted monthly with a mind of its own. And my doctor had taken out my cervix, too, for good measure, and rigged up an artificial vagina by somehow attaching its top somewhere else. Were there bungee cords involved? I didn't know, really, but I knew that I'd never had such pain-free sex ever in my life.

I felt more at home in my body than I'd felt since I was a twelve-year-old, walking alone somewhere in my ripped jeans, thinking my own thoughts. And then, beneath that joy, slowly coming in like a change of weather, I felt a deep relief that brought with it horrific sadness for everyone with a uterus. I realized that the target on my back had been removed.

I didn't really understand how much the weight of that bird's nest had made me afraid, every single day of my life in the country, in this world. I had always known and carried in my uterus the knowledge that it contained the potential to grow my own captivity. The time bomb of one's uterus can be triggered to allow a stranger to change one's life, to alter its course by making one an unwilling parent. I knew this, but I didn't understand it in my body—hadn't understood the humming background noise of fear—until it was gone.

I grew up knowing that getting pregnant could fuck with my access to education, books, work, and freedom. I had experienced the desperation of not being able to afford day care, which I needed to earn money to feed my son, the mobius strip of want that leaves parents completely unprotected in this country, by design, so that we are less free. And I'd felt the million arrows of discrimination and had paid a sort of uterine tax every month before the Affordable Care Act, more expensive insurance because I could grow a child. And all that was gone: my biggest physical vulnerability was gone.

Even without my uterus, I was still a mother. The mothering—all the really hard work—had taken place outside of the uterus, just as my son's amazing next phase of growth is going to take place outside of the nest. The process of mothering changed me, and that is what I want to retain. The nesting and the raising changed this old bird. It must take a fierce patience to turn sticks into a cup.

Mothering made me learn and practice kindness and patience, but also a wily scrappiness and a direct rage at whatever threatened me and my brood. And my mission now is to turn that kindness and patience toward myself, to apply all those skills to my own still-growing life.

I would recommend this emptiness to anyone. I treasure this blankness. My son is fine at college. It's where an eighteen-year-old boy needs to be: out in the world. I'm a tree free of nests, and it is glorious to feel the wind rushing through my branches. I'm a walking tree, I'm a bird considering migration. The explosive and unrestrained uterine energy has been transferred to my entire life, to whatever comes next.

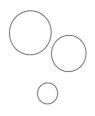

The Antidote

Abigail Thomas

I used to be fond of saying I could get pregnant in an empty room if the radio was tuned to a rock station and something good was playing—the Stones doing "Sweet Virginia," or Leon Russell's "Jumpin' Jack Flash," or any one of hundreds of other songs. I'm an old woman now with an old woman's worries—four children, twelve grandchildren, two great-grandchildren—there's always someone with troubles. I love being old; life is so much simpler, but age doesn't free you from worry—young lives headed into an uncertain future on a planet getting ready to shake us off.

It's been ages since I defined myself by what I looked like or the men I attracted, ages since sex was part of my life, but I still love to get turned on, and rock and roll is still my drug of choice. Talk about a pick-me-up. Consider that moment in the Concert for Bangladesh when George Harrison says, casually, "Coupla numbers from Leon," and then goddamn, there he is, Leon Russell and "Jumpin' Jack Flash," and even at eighty-three, I'm a goner. Who knew lust could be an end in itself? When I was young, this kind of heat was just the beginning. There was always something to be done with it, done about it. But now? It's no longer the means to an end; it is the destination. I'm enjoying the hell out of feeling this alive. "Coupla numbers from Leon," and you better believe that for a little while it's all right, yeah, it's all right now.

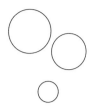

Becoming Your Own Sexual Advocate:
A History of Oppression and the Victories Involving Reproductive Rights

Hillary Leftwich

The Comstock Law of 1873 was enacted in order to restrict any individual from selling or sending what were considered obscenities, including offering any information regarding contraception and abortion. Punishment for violating the law was imprisonment for no less than six months and no more than five years or a fine not less than one hundred dollars and not more than two thousand dollars.

—*Arizona State University,*
The Embryo Project Encyclopedia

I was sixteen when I lost my virginity to my first boyfriend. I was a sophomore in high school, young, doomed, and searching for someone to love me. It didn't matter who it was. David* was the spitting image of Kurt Cobain with bright red hair, and he yielded a skateboard as a weapon. I fell hard and fast for him, and he

---

*Names have been changed in this essay to protect the individual's privacy.

knew it. I lost my virginity in my basement bedroom while the song "Detachable Penis" by King Missile played. I didn't want to have sex, but I did because I didn't want to be a virgin at sixteen. We didn't use a condom. Even if we had one, I was inexperienced and wouldn't know how to put one on. I didn't know if he knew either. The sex education class I took earlier that year was a joke. Boys snickering and making gross comments, while the rest of us were stuck in a state of silence, gaping at enlarged pictures of STD-infested genitals magnified on a screen from a half-busted overhead projector.

> *Planned Parenthood was founded in 1916 by Margaret Sanger, her sister Ethel Byrne, and Fania Mindell. All women were arrested and charged with violating the Comstock Law after providing birth control information from their birth control clinic in Brooklyn, New York. Sanger later opened a clinic in Denver, Colorado, and is still part of the Planned Parenthood of the Rocky Mountains.*
>
> —*Planned Parenthood*

One month later my period was late. My best friend, Sarah, went to the Circle K across the street from our school and bought a pregnancy test with the money from her part-time job. We both worked at the same restaurant, but I used all my money on gas to drive us both to and from school. I sat on the toilet inside a pea-green stall with the words *Fuck Mr. Wright* scrawled in black Sharpie in front of me. Sarah passed the pregnancy test underneath the stall door to me. The sound of my piss splashing against the tip of the pregnancy test only added to the reality of my situation. We both waited for the two lines signifying PREGNANT to appear.

> *In 1979, Planned Parenthood established a national sex education program to ensure teens have access to medically accurate information and confidential health care services. Today, Planned Parenthood is the largest provider of sex education in the country.*
> —*Planned Parenthood*

I was born and raised in the Christian haven city of Colorado Springs under the looming thumb of Dr. James Dobson, founder and former president of Family Talk and Focus on the Family, a nonprofit organization in Colorado Springs that promotes the biblical foundations supporting marriage, family, and child development. Earlier that year, pro-life advocates began gathering in front of different high schools with giant signs of blown-up pictures of aborted fetuses, screaming ABORTION IS A SIN at every high schooler who looked like they had a uterus as they walked or drove by.

> *In 1976 the Hyde Amendment was passed. The law prohibited the use of federal funds to pay for abortion except in extreme cases, such as rape. Studies show when policymakers place severe restrictions on Medicaid coverage of abortion, it forces one in four poor women seeking abortion to carry an unwanted pregnancy to term. Rosie Jimenez, a Latina single mother, was the first woman to die from an illegal abortion after the Hyde Amendment became law.*
> —*Planned Parenthood*

My first encounter with a pro-life, antiabortion group was while I was pulling into the parking lot of my high school. A woman appeared at my passenger window, smashed a photo of a bloody fetus against the glass, and demanded I FOLLOW GOD'S WILL, or I would BURN IN HELL. I honked my horn and told her that if she didn't get the fuck away from my car and the school's private property, I would run her crazy ass over. I meant it. Even at sixteen, I knew my right to an education should not involve escaping a group of antiabortion protestors. After multiple complaints by my school's principal, the protestors scattered to the wind and settled for focusing their shock agenda on Planned Parenthood.

> *In 1973, Roe v. Wade made abortion legal by the decision of the Supreme Court. Since then, according to the National Abortion Federation, data reported from law enforcement agencies across the U.S. pertaining to incidents of violence and disruption against abortion providers from 1977 to 2018 include 11 murders, 26 attempted murders, 42 bombings, 188 arsons, 4,883 trespassing, 100 acid attacks, 663 bioterrorism threats, 290 assault and battery, 664 death threats, four kidnappings, 18,523 hate mail and harassing phone calls, 654 bomb threats, 429,993 picketing, and 6,290 obstruction incidents.*
> —National Abortion Federation

There were rumors around the school surrounding my possible pregnancy. David approached me during lunch and pulled me to the side, away from my friends. He leaned in, his long bangs sweeping across his eyes, his mouth a breath from mine. *If you are what I keep hearing around the school, I'll take care of it myself.* He stepped back and made a pushing motion with his hands. *A fall down the stairs should do it.* I felt a surge of hurt and fear pulse through my body as I watched him walk away, not looking back.

The convenience store pregnancy test I took earlier that day had expired, resulting in what the instructions called an *Inconclusive Result*. The lines could barely be seen. I already knew that if I was pregnant, with the baby of a boy threatening to shove me down a flight of stairs and two more years of high school, I would not continue with the pregnancy.

> *In 1992, in Planned Parenthood Southeastern Pennsylvania v. Casey, the U.S. Supreme Court affirmed a woman's constitutional right to abortion but ruled that states may regulate abortion. This caused a number of states to pass new laws restricting access to abortion.*
>
> —Planned Parenthood

One key figure in the antiabortion movement is Dr. James Dobson. Dobson is clear in his stance on abortion and how it is a sin. Dobson is also clear on his stance about gender identity and same-sex marriage. In 2006, the founder and pastor of New Life Church in Colorado Springs, Ted Haggard, was accused of having sex with a male escort, Mike Jones. Oddly enough, I would find myself, years later, living in the same apartment building as Jones in Denver, and I would have an odd run-in with him when the building caught on fire. He was worried about his memoir going up in flames—the memoir he was writing about his taboo relationship with Haggard. But Dobson supported Haggard, issuing a statement to the media that Haggard's involvement was only a rumor. Haggard later admitted to the affair and underwent conversion therapy. He was fired from New Life Church.

> *The Reverend Tom Davis, an ordained minister with the United Church of Christ, organized clergy across*

> the country in 1994 to mount a theological defense of Planned Parenthood's work. The Clergy Advocacy Board continues to lead a national effort to increase public awareness of the theological and moral bases for advocating reproductive health.
>
> —Planned Parenthood

I needed to know for sure if I was pregnant. It was my first time at a Planned Parenthood, and I was scared shitless. There were no protestors out front, to my relief. The staff was comforting and kind when they led me into an exam room and asked me questions about my sexual history, sexual orientation, and health. My only real experience with sex until that point was the one time with David, which was unprotected. I thought about the STD photos I was shown in sex ed and panicked. The nurse practitioner screening me placed a hand on my shoulder and squeezed. *You're in good hands,* she told me. *We can test you for STDs as well as the pregnancy test.* She handed me a brochure about STDs and another on teen pregnancy and the available options and services. Next, she passed me a small plastic cup and asked me to go to the bathroom. When I was done, I left the cup inside a shelf marked with my name and date of birth in the bathroom and returned to the exam room. While I waited, I read the brochures the nurse gave me. I was scared, worried, and nervous, but knowing I had options and a place to go for help was comforting. Five minutes later, the nurse returned to the exam room, shut the door, and stared at the clipboard in her hands. I held my breath, positive that she could hear my heart pounding.

> *In response to many black women being denied access to health and social services at the height of the Depression, the New York Urban League endorsed Margaret*

> *Sanger's new Harlem clinic. In 1932, Dr. N. Louise Young, the first black woman to practice medicine in Maryland, opened her practice in Baltimore and later oversaw a Planned Parenthood center with assistance from the Urban League.*
>
> —Planned Parenthood

My pregnancy test came back negative. Was I lucky? Yes. I felt stupid, uneducated about sex, and angry that I bore the burden of responsibility if I had become pregnant. David would not have provided any type of support, including financial, had I chosen to keep the baby or if I had decided to get an abortion. My experience as a teenager with pregnancy scares didn't end with my first incident. Sex as a teenager is never planned, never convenient, and doesn't always involve protection. Sexual education in school was a joke. The information I received was outdated and involved statistics from the 1970s. I didn't know all my options for birth control. I didn't know that sexual assault should be taken seriously.

> *Among adult women an estimated 32,101 pregnancies result from rape each year. Among 34 cases of rape-related pregnancy, the majority occurred among adolescents and resulted from assault by a known, often related perpetrator. Only 11.7% of these victims received immediate medical attention after the assault, and 47.1% received no medical attention related to the rape. A total 32.4% of these victims did not discover they were pregnant until they had already entered the second trimester.*
>
> —American Journal of Obstetrics and Gynecology

Even after my first time with David and my pregnancy scare, I continued an on-again, off-again relationship with him. One time, during sex, I asked him to stop, but he kept going, crying, as he pushed himself on me. I remained silent, not knowing if it was rape because I consented to have sex with him. This wouldn't be my first or last experience; there would be a traumatizing series of unwanted sexual contact as well as assaults, including my friends' experiences with sexual assault, hate crime attacks, trying to navigate their own sexual identities, and desperately needing a support system in a time when LGBTQ rights were a source of national attention in my home state. In 1992, Colorado became known as "The Hate State." Religious fundamentalists rooted mainly in Colorado Springs wrote a measure known as Amendment 2 to amend the state's constitution, which prevented legislative, executive, or judicial action from recognizing homosexuals or bisexuals as a protected class. The amendment was approved by a vote of 53 percent to 47 percent. It was later struck down in 1996 by the United States Supreme Court (*Colorado Encyclopedia*, "Amendment 2").

> *If the U.S. Supreme Court had accepted Amendment 2, it would have meant an end to the recent rash of anti-gay initiatives that tried to change the rules. Moreover, it would have prevented this kind of device from being used against any other minority in the future (it had been used once in the past, against African Americans in the 1960s).*
> —*American Civil Liberties Union*

When I was sixteen, I needed access to serious, up-to-date sex education and birth control options. I needed to know that as a woman twenty years later, the sex I experienced as a teenager and the sex I experience as an adult would have similarities and differences. Sex with a woman doesn't always mean someone is a lesbian, and sex with a man doesn't mean someone is straight. Gender identity and sexual orientation are not always connected, and it shouldn't be society's business to try to define this. Orgasms aren't just for men. It's okay to say no or stop, even after you have started. Sometimes, the safest, most enjoyable sex you can have is with yourself. Sex and all the different ways it can happen and who it happens with is not something to be ashamed of. A healthy, trusting sexual relationship should be something everyone experiences. But it's not. It took almost twenty-five years for me to find a partner I feel safe and comfortable with. To find the trust not only to explore each other's bodies but also to have fun. To bond and form the most intimate of connections. Sex shouldn't be about losing your virginity or doing it to find love. Having support and knowledge from trusted organizations and people who can educate us to make the best decision for our bodies and lives is invaluable. Teenagers will not become safe, protected adults and advocates for their bodies and boundaries unless they have this support. Sometimes advocating for ourselves takes a lifetime to learn. And most times, the learning never stops.

References

American Civil Liberties Union (ACLU), "Preview of 1995 Court Term: Lesbian and Gay Rights," 1995, https://www.aclu.org/press-releases/preview-1995-court-term-lesbian-and-gay-rights.

Arizona State University, "The Comstock Law (1873)," *The Embryo Project Encyclopedia*, 2018, https://embryo.asu.edu/pages/comstock-law-1873.

M. M. Holmes, H. S. Resnick, D. G. Kilpatrick, and C. L. Best, "Rape-Related Pregnancy: Estimates and Descriptive Characteristics from a National Sample of Women," *American Journal of Obstetrics and Gynecology* 175, no. 2 (August 1996): 320–4, https://doi.org/10.1016/S0002-9378(96)70141-2.

Planned Parenthood, "Planned Parenthood Is 100 Years Strong," October 11, 2016, https://www.plannedparenthood.org/about-us/newsroom/press-releases/planned-parenthood-is-100-years-strong.

National Abortion Federation, "2018 Violence and Disruption Statistics," https://prochoice.org/wp-content/uploads/2018-Anti-Abortion-Violence-and-Disruption.pdf.

Richard Ramirez, "Amendment 2," *Colorado Encyclopedia*, last modified March 30, 2023, https://coloradoencyclopedia.org/article/amendment-2.

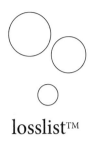

losslist™

Sarah Swandell

Having a miscarriage shower? losslist™ is the one-stop shop for all you need!

container for passed tissue
Not to be confused with snack-size containers typically housing almonds or baby carrots, this custom cube is perfect for hiding your specimen until you are ready to show it to your husband, who will suggest putting it in the fridge in case the doctor wants to see. (The doctor will not want to see.)
price: $2.19 for a pack of six
quantity: single

take-out food
Especially necessary for your first dinner after the appointment, with a plethora of choices to suit your empty appetite. Please note, burgers will be cooked to order; we suggest you wait by taking a walk around the darkened block. When your food is ready, we'll call you from a random local number, which you will believe, with the sweetest, blindest pilgrim faith, is the doctor's office, calling at 6:37 in the evening (as doctor's offices are wont

to do) to say, "Ma'am, we're so sorry, but your file got mixed up. Your hCG levels look good; the pregnancy is still viable." All the better since you'd already planned not to have alcohol with your meal, just in case.
price: $15–$18/meal, plus tax and tip
quantity: unlimited

grocery-store flowers (assorted)
Fresh and fragrance-free! These long stems from your husband, brought home on day three of bleeding, will keep in the refrigerator an additional sixteen days until you are ready to take them, along with the specimen (also in the refrigerator), out to the backyard to bury. The jewel tones of these petals will be the perfect contrast to the February that surrounds you as you sit on a cold bench and say dumb prayers and snot your way through reading a letter to your baby. (Even you, ever protective of your grief, will wonder whether this is slightly ridiculous. The yellow spikes of the flowers will beam up at you from the hole in the soil as you mentally vacillate between daring anyone to judge you and judging yourself for the lunacy of burying tiny tissue while reading aloud sentiments like "Thank you for making me a mother.")
price: $12.99
quantity: one bouquet

lingerie set
This bright, lacy little number is perfect for being intimate with your husband—though not with actual intercourse, of course, as the doctor forbids it until the bleeding stops. No matter! Don this duo of halter-top bra and peek-a-boo panties, and you'll prove to your husband and yourself and the world that everything is fine!
** *Insider tip:* This item is best ordered in red, or afterward it will reveal a few drops of blood, which last through several wash-

ings, and every time you see it in your drawer, you'll wonder why you don't just throw it out.
price: $24.99
quantity: one matching set in selected color (peach)

errands-runner
Every new-loss mom could use a trusty sidekick to tackle all her exhausting errands! Need to return books you've barely begun? Why drive to the library yourself? Let your errands-runner drop off *The Pregnancy Encyclopedia*, *The Pregnancy Bible*, and *The Official Lamaze Guide: Giving Birth with Confidence*. Have a sudden urge to burn the black and red sweater you were wearing during those eight hours in the ER? Your errands-runner will gladly pop over to Goodwill and even pick up a charity donation tax form.

** *Optional upgrade to a personal assistant* who will white-out the calendar entry that says "prenatal appt. 3:15!" with three hearts beside it (for the new family of three!); unsubscribe you from your What to Expect, Pregnancy+, CineMama, and The Bump apps; and, on your Life app, click "end pregnancy."

price: $15–$20/hour, unless you enlist a friend . . . but surely you can do it yourself?
quantity: N/A

wall décor that says "There is always always always something to be thankful for"
Which your pastor John will reference as you sit crying in front of him. This cheery wooden sign hangs in the kitchen of Kathryn, a fellow church member. "Think of Kathryn's sign," John will say, John with his two living children and his second home on the coast: "There is always always always something to be thankful for." It has been ten days since the death, and new tears are being

added to your face this very moment, and he is looking at you with always always always.
price: $95.00 for 16x20 canvas
quantity: fuck

Neiman Marcus cookies in a green-and-gold striped bag
A hearty blend of ground oats, thick butter, milk chocolate chips, and 4 oz. finely grated dark chocolate, this comfort-food classic lives up to its deluxe name. Nothing will minister to you as these round blessings do. Nothing will get you out of bed except a trip to the kitchen, where your reward awaits. You will be so grateful to the coworker who left these cookies on your desk, you won't get rid of the gift bag for the next four years.
price: $250 for the recipe, according to legend
quantity: two dozen, eaten over two days

texts from a friend, just to check in
Designed to be sent immediately after the loss, but also after a couple weeks have passed, and also after everyone else has stopped asking how you are, like even three months after the loss, and even when you are pregnant with your rainbow baby—which is helpful, because you will still listen to P!nk's "Beam Me Up" and cry over the lost baby at the same time the living baby kicks gleefully and determinedly for your attention.
  ** *Special feature:* These texts will come from a woman who not only has never had a miscarriage; she's never had children. Which makes you marvel, all the more grateful, that somehow she gets it.
price: standard messaging rates apply
quantity: more than you expected, which turns out to be the right amount

walk with a friend
For an unlimited time, this gift will take your miscarriage registry to the next level. Join Kathryn on a walk through the sandhills of Nick's Creek Greenway to talk about nothing but grief, with which she is familiar since she and her husband discovered their son cold after an overdose in his bedroom one Easter morning. He was nineteen. "Life is not solid," she will say. "It's shaky and mysterious. It's been this way all along. You just didn't know it." And you will go home and write down everything she says so you don't forget. She won't say, *There is always always always something to be thankful for.* She will say, *You can be grateful to the person you lost—grateful for what they taught you through this. The lessons will* never *be more valuable than they are. But they're something to hold on to.*

** *Bonus content:* This walk includes Kathryn's practical advice for what to do when someone says, "I know you know God has a plan." One gracious way to respond, instead of calling them a dumbfuck, is: "I appreciate you trying to be helpful, but that's not where I am right now."

** *Not included:* Any pointing out of the difference between her loss of a teenage son and your loss of a seven-week-old embryo.

** *Complimentary add-on:* She will ask what name you chose for your child, and she will use that name every time she brings him up, ever since. You will go home cleansed, and she will go home to her kitchen to look at the hanging wooden wall décor.

price: 90 minutes of an afternoon
quantity: unquantifiable

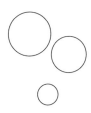

An Imagined Conversation with My Local School District in Which I Advocate for Heavily Menstruating Students

Joy Victory

Austin Independent School District parent announcement: "All prescription and nonprescription medications will now require medical orders from providers and parental consent for student use/administration on campus."

Me: Wait, really? What about ibuprofen?

District: Even ibuprofen.

Me: Why?

District: It's a medication.

Me: So?

District: Medications . . . do things. Kids can . . . use them. To . . . do things.

Me: Huh?

District: Bad things. With bad outcomes.

Me: With ibuprofen!?

District: Yes. It's better to be safe than sorry.

Me: *Dude.* Have you ever had a period?

District: What does that have to do with our medication policy? We do everything in the interest of student safety and learning.

Me: I should hope so. But this could do more harm than good. I think I'm going to have to be more blunt about this. I know! Got time for a quick story? It's about a girl. A girl named . . .

District: Wait! Is she a student in our district? Has she signed a release form?

Me (rolls eyes): No. The girl is a composite—you know, drawn from the nightmares I still have about being a female teen.

District: Oh. I guess that's okay, then. (Checks phone.) We'll give you five minutes, but then we've got a meeting to discuss district employee pay raises.

Me: This will be quick, I promise. Our story begins in a high school biology classroom in a midsize Texas city. A teen girl (totally coincidentally) named Joy has just gotten her period. From the heavy, wet plop that landed on her underwear, she could tell it was going to be a doozy, one of those periods that would make her feel faint . . .

District (looks ill): Oh no.

Me: Ha! I'm just getting started. Joy needed the bathroom *now*, but with ten minutes to go until class ended, she knew her teacher would say no. It had happened before. To cope, Joy whispered her mantra, one she will say monthly for the next few decades of her life until she can't take it anymore and has surgery:

Please don't bleed through. Please don't bleed through. Please don't bleed through.

District (cringes, looks a little faint): Uhh . . .

Me: Stay with me. When the bell rang, Joy rushed to the bathroom and ran into the nearest stall. Only a little bit had leaked onto her jeans. *Whew.* Her relief was brief, though, because she had a new, even grosser problem: no toilet paper and no trash can in the stall! Fuck. Joy stared at the floor for far too long, paralyzed with shame. Sometimes, when she had no other choice, she'd leave her partially wrapped "feminine products" on the floor. Along with her dignity. Fortunately, another student eventually passed her some under the stall.

District: Dignity?

Me: . . .

District: Oh, right, toilet paper.

Me: The only bright spot in this tragic bloodbath was that Joy had ibuprofen in her backpack. Her "magic pills." The nickname was fitting because one day it would be revealed in medical research that ibuprofen really is magic, *especially* for periods!

District (looks skeptical): Magic?

Me: Yes! Okay, technically not magic. Scientists learned that ibuprofen inhibits prostaglandins, these bitchy little hormone-like chemicals that go apeshit and wreak havoc on the uterus. Two tablets of ibuprofen not only made Joy feel better; she bled a lot less . . . and . . . well . . . um . . .

District: Yes?

Me: There's another hellish thing prostaglandins do. It's hard to say out loud. It's like, *good god*.

District: ?

Me (mumbles): They stop the "period poops."

District (eyes widen in both horror and curiosity): Period poops!?

Me: Yeah. Loose stool, diarrhea, the squirts, bubble guts, pooplear explosions. You haven't lived until you've been in a poorly stocked school bathroom with a trifecta of body fluids streaming out of you.

District: This is making me want ibuprofen and I don't even have a uterus.

Me: That's the magic of storytelling! But listen, before Joy could swallow her magic pills, a teacher walked in. "What is that? Are those drugs?" barked the teacher, who apparently was blessed with only light-flow days. "You know it's against school policy!"

Overly compliant to authority figures, Joy placed them in the teacher's hand. Then she fled to a different stall, this time choosing one with adequate toilet paper, because she not only had more period poops to contend with, but also her tears—

District: Okay. Okay. Okay. We get it. But as we stated, we're not banning medication. We're saying children must get their parents to give consent, and then parents must get their doctor to give orders for ANY medication. And then, once that's done, whenever a student needs it, ta-da!

Me: Where? In the nurse's office?

District: Yes, for safety reasons, of course.

Me: So, a girl must ask whatever teacher is around if she can have a nurse's pass, and when the teacher asks why, she must explain she has her period and she would like some ibuprofen, and while she does this, both of them blush, the teacher feeling sorry for the girl yet also squeamish . . . and the girl feeling humiliated?

District: (nods tentatively).

Me: And then, after that, she has to wait for the nurse to "administer" it to her? Meanwhile, the girl is bleeding with a horrible case of the runs, and, because this all takes so damn long, she's missing a critical lesson on mitosis, meaning she may never fulfill her dream of becoming a geneticist?

District: That's one way of putting it! But yes. Medications can do things. Kids can use them: We can't allow students to carry ibuprofen when it could be a gateway drug to OxyContin.

Me: Has that been a problem?

District: Theoretically? Yes. Literally? No. But . . . (checks phone). Oh wow, gotta run!

Me: Wait, I'm not done . . . (looks down as phone buzzes. District seizes opportunity and runs off. The phone call is from . . . the district?)

District voice message: *Thank you for listening and sending your scholar to an AISD school! Should you need further assistance, please message us via the Student Services system. Response time ranges from two days to two years, depending on call volume and general interest levels. Have a fabulous day!*

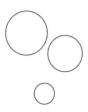

Barren: A Journey

Alyse Knorr

A large black cardboard box, the size of a five-year-old, sits propped up in the back seat of our car, buckled securely in place by both lap and shoulder belts. "KEEP UPRIGHT" reads the bold red sticker on the side of the box. "THIS END UP." "DO NOT DROP." This is the first photo ever taken of my son, and this is the story of how he came to be.

The plan my wife, Kate, and I made was quintessentially feminist—a cliché of lesbian family-making. Kate would have our first child, and I would have our second. Two uteruses, two pregnancies, two childbirths. Fair is fair. We would literally share the labor of labor. Conceiving our older daughter was fast. Kate got pregnant after only one IUI, aka intrauterine insemination—the standard clinical procedure for lesbian couples. We had steeled ourselves for many failed attempts and much heartache and stress, but we faced none of those—not with Kate, at least.

My pregnancy attempts failed entirely. I passed all the fertility tests with flying colors, but after six failed IUIs (including one two-day chemical pregnancy that filled me with hope, then broke my heart), the doctors had no explanation for why I couldn't conceive. I was as confused as they were. In my mind, an IUI was so straightforward—inserting sperm directly into the uterus during ovulation—that it seemed impossible it *couldn't* work. It was as if eighty million men had been deposited at the front door of a woman's house at the exact time she was guaranteed to be home, but not a single man knocked on her door. The best explanation the doctors could give me was that it was just plain old bad luck.

After my eighth failed IUI, we decided to try IVF. And after purchasing $6,000 of IVF drugs and then realizing after the first round of injections that I am violently allergic to IVF drugs, I made the painful decision to give up on ever carrying a child. Kate—who had already given away her old maternity clothes after our daughter was born and looked forward to a life of never having to be pregnant again—heroically offered to carry our second child. But she wanted to use a different fertility clinic than the one I had used. Which left us with a new mission: transporting our donor sperm from my clinic to hers.

And so we showed up one cold winter day at a tall brick building full of suspicious-looking medical offices ("Spine Clinic," "Expert Laser Treatment," "Jonathan Lee Hormones and Anti-Aging Aesthetics") to rent a cryotank from a company whose name I'll charitably change to CryoSolutions. Let me be clear that we did not choose CryoSolutions. CryoSolutions was the only game in town. I think they knew this, too. Their website, which looked like it was made on GeoCities, could have tipped us off to the situation—or the brochure, which looked like their son made it on PowerPoint fifteen years ago and which featured an enormous picture of a single sperm on the front. "Cryotank rental, cryopreservation, fertility testing, and anonymous donor sperm for purchase," the inside read. "Long-term storage of sperm, oocytes, and embryos."

When we opened the door to the CryoSolutions office, we found a man in his sixties, wearing jeans and a plaid shirt, sitting at a flimsy IKEA desk. The floors of the cramped room were covered in old tan carpet, and the air smelled like a bad hotel. The room was full of a chaotic jumble of tacky home décor and clutter, lending the energy of a grandparent's home office. An enormous clock from Marshall's hung on one wall and a deer-hunting calendar on another. In one corner stood a mini fridge with a sleeve of Solo cups beside it, along with a haphazard pile of cocoa packets. In another corner of the room, a shaky-looking end table sported an ancient desktop printer, several spray bottles of disinfectant, and a bowl full of empty sperm vials the size of ChapStick containers.

The man at the desk opened up a crusty binder full of old papers. He asked us to sign in on a printed Excel spreadsheet and then nodded at the cryotanks, which stood unceremoniously out on the floor, each in a three-foot-tall black cardboard box.

"Have you ever used one of these before?" he asked.

"Of course not," I wanted to say, but just shook my head instead. At this point, I was utterly shocked at the disarray of the room. I suppose I was expecting something that looked like Star Trek—or at least vaguely sterile enough to house human embryos—but this room made our conversation feel like an illicit Craigslist transaction.

The man said nothing, but got up and walked to the other side of the room to the "lab," which resembled an office break room. In the lab, an older woman was using a pipette to suck up specimens from cups and deposit them into vials. The man ducked into the kitchen, put his hand on the woman's shoulder, and murmured a question to her. *Ah*, I thought—*so this is a mom-and-pop operation. A mom-and-pop sperm shop.*

"When should we bring this back?" Kate asked after the man returned and lugged a tank over for us.

"How's next Tuesday?" he asked.

Next Tuesday! I thought. *I'm moving the sperm today—I don't want this tank for an entire week!*

"What do we do with it for the week?" Kate said, reading my mind. The man looked confused by the question. "Where should we keep it?" she tried. His face stayed blank, eyebrows raised. "There's some sort of freezing mechanism, right?" Kate asked, flustered. "Do we need to worry about keeping it somewhere cold?"

We did not. We gave the man $150, and he gave us the tank. He provided no instructions whatsoever for how to use or care for the tank. We didn't sign any kind of liability waiver to rent this very expensive piece of equipment. We provided no collateral. We made no promises not to throw the tank off a bridge or transport human organs in it. The man just handed us the tank like it was a beer cooler, and we left Mom and Pop to their sperm work.

We each took one end of the box and carried the heavy tank down the hallway. We entered the elevator, alone, on the sixth floor. On the fourth floor, the elevator doors opened to a tall man in his fifties who raised an eyebrow at us.

"Can I . . . join you all?" he asked. We nodded and he entered the elevator. We waited in awkward silence for several seconds while he stared pointedly at the tank. *He's going to ask*, I thought. *It's inevitable. There's no way around it.*

"What's the box for?" he finally asked.

"Sperm," I answered, before he'd even finished the question.

"Wow," he said, blinking at the enormous box. "That's a lot of sperm."

"It's actually empty now," I said. "But when it's full, it'll only be like this much," I added, gesturing with my thumb and index finger. The man nodded gravely, then cast his eyes away, unsettled to have received more than he bargained for in this conversation.

I should have been used to it by now—the stares, the invasive questions. Going through infertility treatment is an exercise in humiliation. Doctors and nurses look straight through you, seeing only the size of your follicles or the number on your hCG test. If you're over thirty-five, you're a "geriatric mother," and after four failed IUIs, you're re-classified from "normal lesbian trying to get knocked up" to "patient with unexplained infertility." Before we could undergo our first IUI, Kate and I had to be screened by a psychologist to make sure we were fit for conceiving with donor sperm—to make sure we wouldn't tell our future kid crazy lies about her origins.

The atmosphere at my old fertility clinic was exactly the opposite of CryoSolutions. The waiting room was slick and sleek—all gleaming, shiny glass, immaculate laminate floors, and hip spaceship-style chairs. As we waited beside a $1,000 espresso machine at the empty desk for a receptionist to appear, a fertility doctor who had subjected me to an unnecessary outpatient procedure passed by.

"Do you ladies need any help?" he asked.

You don't remember me? I wanted to ask him. *You roughed up my uterine lining during a sonohysterogram and then sent me to the hospital for a hysteroscopy to check out the suspicious spot you yourself created.* I will never forget the feeling of waking up from the anesthesia and noticing, with bewilderment, that I was wearing a pair of gauzy medical underwear. No one had warned me I'd wake up in a different pair of underwear.

We were ushered downstairs to the andrology lab to pick up our sperm. The andrology lab consisted of a sliding glass window and a hallway to two small private rooms. The door to one of the rooms was open, and I craned my neck to peek inside. The lights were turned down low, but I could still make out an armchair, a sink, and a TV with lots of porn loaded up.

"That must be where the guys jack off," I said far too loudly to Kate, who elbowed me.

I frowned, thinking wistfully about how much more pleasant certain steps in this process must be for male parents-to-be than for female. Of course, infertility is painful for everyone involved. But I doubt many male patients experience lows like the one I had around IUI number four, when I winced and gasped on the table while the doctor tried and repeatedly failed to insert a catheter into my uterus. "This shouldn't be painful," he chastised, frustrated at me for my squirming and moans of pain. It felt like he was jabbing at my cervix with a plastic fork.

Just then, an older woman in blue scrubs popped her head out of the sliding glass window, which reminded me of a McDonald's drive-thru.

"Can I help you?" she asked in a cheerful voice.

"We're here to transport our sperm," Kate said.

The woman nodded and handed us some forms to fill out. "DO NOT LEAVE SPECIMENS UNATTENDED," read a sign over the sliding glass window. I looked at the woman, grinning eagerly, and wanted desperately to ask her how she got into this line of work. *This is her career,* I thought. *She accepts and ships out deliveries of frozen sperm. She counts sperm under a microscope all day long.* And I could tell, by the stuffed-animal sperm next to her computer's mouse pad, that she must really love her job.

Despite all my frustrations with the IUI process, I understood an appreciation—or even affection—for sperm. Sperm share some of the qualities that I like most about myself: They're hardworking, determined, and brave. Also often bad at directions. I felt such a fondness for sperm that I had even taken to calling our imaginary second child "Tad," as in "tadpole," since that is what sperm look like. I always viewed the insemination process as a team effort, and so, about thirty minutes before each procedure, when the andrology lab would call to get my verbal consent to thaw and prepare the sperm, I would always offer them my encouragement. "Wish them good luck for me!" I would tell the andrology lab—perhaps this very woman.

Kate and I signed the stack of papers about who would be driving the sperm and to what address, whom the sperm currently belonged to, and who was "gifting" it to whom. That's the term the forms used—*gifting*.

"You're welcome, babe," I whispered to Kate, who was not having any of my shit.

"You are aware," the lab technician said soberly, "that you need to leave your windows cracked in the car while you drive this over, correct?"

I resisted finding something to joke about, and Kate shook her head.

"Nitrogen displaces oxygen," the woman said. "If you don't crack your windows, you could pass out on the drive over."

"The sperm could kill us?" I blurted out.

"Did CryoSolutions not tell you this?" she asked.

Of course not. Of course CryoSolutions did not tell us this crucial piece of information about their equipment.

Satisfied with our safety preparation, the lab tech disappeared to find our sperm and put it in the tank.

"It's like this lady's running a nuclear submarine," Kate whispered, and I was glad she was starting to lighten up. The truth is that utter frankness and dark humor had carried me through my infertility struggles, distracting me from my heartbreak and allowing me to reroute a fraction of my despair. A friend recently told me that shortly after she met me, she asked how I was doing, and I replied, "I could be better, honestly. Trying to get pregnant, but I've got bad luck and a bad womb." Infertility is supposed to be a private, taboo topic never to be spoken of. By talking so openly about it, I threw off the mantle of shame and insisted that those around me keep me company in my discomfort. I still make jokes about it now: about how useless my period is, or that the reason I'm barren—yes, that's the word I prefer, because it matches my biblical level of sorrow about the situation—is because I'm so gay that sperm die as soon as they enter my body. Humor—even very bad jokes like this one—has always helped me.

The woman returned with our sperm all tucked into the cryotank, and we left triumphantly to begin the last leg of our journey—the trip to Kate's clinic, where we would hopefully conceive our second child.

Outside in the parking lot, we buckled the box up in the back seat, and just like that, half of our future child was in the front seat, inside of my wife, and the other half was in the back. I marveled at this—how all the parts of a new person could exist, contained in the car just a few feet away from each other. The sperm and the egg. All our hopes and dreams. The sadness, the pain, the humor, the joy. It's only when you mix them together that you get the miracle: my son, who is sixteen months old as of this writing and the universe's perfect answer to the question "Why me?" *Lucky you. Lucky, lucky, wildly lucky you.*

We turned on our "Baby" playlist—a collection of songs with "Baby" in the title, like the Ronettes' "Be My Baby" and Britney Spears's ". . . Baby One More Time." We made the playlist back when we were working to conceive our daughter, and it was our tradition to play it as we traveled to and from every fertility clinic appointment. On this trip, I immediately turned on the extremely appropriate "Ice, Ice, Baby," and Kate and I laughed and laughed.

We drove the sperm across the city. Late morning sunrise gleamed off the skyscrapers downtown, casting a golden glow on the road ahead of us.

"Welcome to Denver, Tad," Kate said.

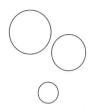

Hold On, It's a Rough Ride

Angelique Fawns

I'm leaning against the rail in the indoor arena at the fairgrounds watching equine speed events. The horses are kicking up dirt, which tickles my nostrils and makes my eyes water. The rock-country music is blaring so loud it makes me wince. When I was younger, I used to compete. Now I'm a fifty-year-old spectator. Though my fingers twitch and I'm leaning into the turns with the riders, I'm not saddling up. My joints hurt, and I'm afraid of falling.

Hit the ground when you are twenty, you bounce. Hit it after forty, you break.

Dust swirls by the bleachers, mixing with the cool spring air billowing through the entrance. Crossing my fingers, I take a deep breath of hay, leather, and livestock. A new song comes on, something by a new singer called Jelly Bean, or Jelly Roll, or something that sounds like a dessert, and my hips shake to the beat.

I stop dancing when my daughter roars into the ring, her long blond hair streaming behind her, and the horse flying at a breakneck speed.

In the wrong direction.

They are supposed to be weaving through a set of six poles, but instead, they are galloping around the bottom of the arena. The horse won't even start the pattern.

Faith struggles with the sweaty, furious horse. We call the mare Crazy Pants, and she is living up to her name. She is shaking her head and bucking like she's auditioning for a rodeo bronc.

Her coach, an intense horsewoman in a cowboy hat, is standing by the gate. "Loosen her reins and give her a kick," she says.

I clap my hands and add encouragement. "Get her up there! You can do it."

Faith scowls at me and then concentrates on her pattern. Each pole is twenty-one feet apart. Competitors are supposed to run their horses to the top of the ring, weave through the poles, and then turn around and weave back up them.

Sweat trickles down my temple as I pray the horse will listen to her. After what feels like hours, but is only a few minutes, Faith manages to weave her horse through the poles one way, but Crazy Pants quits when she gets near the chute—the place the horses run through to enter the arena.

My daughter is being dragged out of the ring.

Faith begs Crazy Pants to move by throwing the reins up by her ears and giving her a series of swift kicks.

The mare stops. Now she won't move at all.

Faith changes tactics and decides to comfort her horse rather than insist on finishing the pattern. With a soothing pat, they walk out of the ring.

"No time for Crazy Pants this round," the announcer's voice calls out over the loudspeakers.

My face turns bright red, and my core temperature goes up about five degrees. My bra is instantly drenched as nausea fills my mouth with saliva.

This isn't a reaction to Faith's disastrous pole performance.

This has been happening to me approximately twenty times a day for the last several months.

I would give anything just to feel normal again.

It takes a few minutes, but the feeling of burning alive subsides. With a shuddering breath, I walk out of the arena and catch up with my daughter taking her horse back to her stall.

It's only a short walk, but I must hustle to catch up to my daughter.

Faith whirls on me, pulling her horse to a halt. "Mom, why were you yelling? I know I had to get her through the pattern. You totally embarrassed me."

I stop on the concrete path in shock. My insides turn to ice, my hands tremble, and tears fill my eyes.

"I just wanted to help," I say.

Faith's jaw drops when she notices tears streaming down my face. "Are you okay, Mom? It's okay that you yelled at me. I'm sorry." Her horse nudges her with a sweaty nose and yanks. "I have to take Crazy back to her stall before she runs me over, but I'm really sorry."

She's a sweet kid and would never deliberately hurt my feelings. I know that. It's logical that she would be upset if her young, green horse misbehaved.

Faith's high-strung mare pulls her away, and I'm not just crying now. I am ugly-bawling. Putting a hand over my face, I rush to the side of the barn and fall to my knees on the grass. Luckily there is no one in this area.

I clench my fists and try to regain control. "Count to ten. You're going to be okay." I manage to calm myself down. My eyes are still filled with tears, but at least snot isn't running down my face anymore.

What the hell is happening to me?

Past me would have threatened to bring pom-poms to Faith's next event.

"You think I'm embarrassing you? That was nothing. Wait till I wear a cheer uniform and wave these around."

When I hit fifty, I hit menopause.

The hot flashes, new mustache, and extra chin were unpleasant, but these random crying jags? Untenable.

Back home, I book an appointment with my nurse practitioner. Hers is a small, friendly office with twenty-year-old décor and intimate examination rooms.

"I need something to help me with my hormones and these unbearable hot flashes," I say.

She is a young practitioner. "It is a normal passage of life. You will get through it." Her long, dark hair is caught in a ponytail, and she consults my medical records. "Your latest blood test was normal, but your cholesterol is a bit high."

I clench my hands in my lap and try again. "My cholesterol isn't giving me hot flashes. I've heard of hormone therapy. There must be something I can do to help with this."

She frowns. "Studies have shown that estrogen affects your heart and blood vessels. I'm not comfortable prescribing hormone replacement. It increases your risk of clots and a heart attack."

Sweat pours down the sides of my face. I feel as if the devil just grabbed me in a hug. "See! I'm having a hot flash right now. There must be something."

She looks at my red cheeks and taps her fingers on her desk. "There is something called Effexor. It's an antidepressant, and it can also work to help control vasomotor symptoms. Like hot flashes. Would you like to try that?"

I blink. "An antidepressant? But I'm not depressed. I might cry more, but most of the time my mood is fine."

"They've had some great success with it, and there is less cardiovascular risk."

"So let me get this straight. You are willing to give me something that will alter my brain chemicals to fix my hormone issues? I'm not comfortable with screwing with my brain chemistry."

I left the office perplexed. For the next few months, I suffer:

When my husband or daughter says something insensitive, I bawl.

Night sweats make me change my sheets—every damn day.

I find someone who can wax a mustache.

Even in an air-conditioned office, I turn a big fan on several times a day to avoid being barbecued in my skin.

Finally, the ultimate injustice: My big toe turns yellow with a fungal infection. Google lets me know this could be because my feet sweat all night.

Back to the doctor's office:

This time there is a new nurse practitioner. She gives me something for my toe, and I tell her about my symptoms. Her mother suffered horribly from menopause, and hormone replacement was her salvation.

"Why suffer? Let's start hormone therapy immediately," she says.

Cue the heavens opening and angels singing. I start a regime of estrogen and progesterone.

***

A few months later, I'm back at the fairgrounds.

This time I am sitting on a horse waiting to compete. Icy rain is falling outside, but the arena is warm. I stroke the neck of my big black mare and smile at Faith. She has just run a lovely barrel pattern on Crazy Pants. A bit more coaching was the answer.

My daughter's eyes sparkle with excitement. "Crazy Pants loves the barrels. I'm so glad we decided not to do poles with her." She leaves the arena on her prancing horse.

Nerves toss my belly, like the endless salads I eat. Not that I could stomach breakfast today. I am too nervous. My cheeks are flushed and my heart is thumping. It feels wonderful.

"On deck, we have Boo," the announcer says.

With a cluck, I send my horse down the chute and into the ring. I point her toward the first barrel and lean back for the turn. Sweat dampens my plaid shirt, but not from a hot flash. I haven't had one of those for ages.

"Go Mom!" Faith says from the sidelines. "You got this."

Grabbing onto the horn, I haul my body out of the saddle and send Boo for the second barrel. My joints creak a little, but I keep up with her lunge. My heart is pumping with adrenaline, and I feel a bloom of warmth in my chest.

I feel alive. Young.

We turn the second as I grit my teeth and head for the third. Boo is getting a little tired, so I squeeze my calves to keep her going. The smell of her warm body and creak of my saddle are familiar and pleasant. We turn the final barrel and gallop home. I can feel the grin stretching my face from ear to ear as I trip the timer and we finish the run.

We don't win, but I do feel like a winner.

Hormone therapy has made my joints feel better, given me back my emotional control, and stopped those devilish hot flashes. Women shouldn't have to suffer if they don't have to. Even if they're fifty.

It's not time to hang up my spurs just yet.

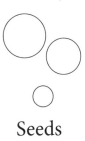

Seeds

Yoda Olinyk

A nurse pushes me down a barren hallway toward the exit. I am not leaving through the back door masked in secrecy, like the other women who are being discharged from the clinic today. At first, this wheelchair feels excessive, but my attempt to stand makes me feel like a newborn fawn on ice. The nurse's cheeks are fixed with a permanent half smile, and she assures me again that this is normal. She hands me some pamphlets and my appointment card for my follow-up appointment. The nurse delivers me to my best friend, who is both awkward and brave when helping me into my car. My best friend is new to this grief of mine, too, and doesn't say a word as I sob the whole car ride back. I wish we were driving home, but we are going back to the Airbnb I rented so that I could rest for a few nights before I had to make the three-day road trip back home. My best friend flew across the country to make the drive with me, but at this moment, I do not thank her. I do not say a word to her until the next morning, when I crawl out of bed in a grief-mangled stupor and tell her that I think something is wrong.

My best friend consults the pamphlet given at the hospital. It states that abdominal pain and bleeding after an abortion are normal. Both the pamphlet and Google give the same sanguineous warning: Go to the emergency department if the bleeding exceeds one maxi pad in less than an hour. So I put a fresh pad in my underwear, and we wait. I surge with hunger pangs after two weeks of fierce morning sickness, so my best friend makes me a comically large bowl of buttered noodles for breakfast and sits with me in the sunroom as I wolf them down and ask for seconds. She treads lightly while attending to my needs. She brings me tea and juice. She asks questions without asking too much. She holds my hand, holds my hair back, and holds my grief for the next several days until I am well enough to start the long drive home.

My cramping worsens, but I don't go to the emergency department. My best friend buys maxi pads at every pit stop. We spend the night in a beach town, take a rainy walk, and catch a sunset. We watch a Bette Midler movie marathon—the only thing playing on the retro TV at our roadside motel—and my best friend pauses and fast-forwards anytime there is mention of a baby or a pregnancy. She does this at every motel we stop at for the next two days. A few days later, my best friend tucks me into my own bed before she flies home. Tells me to call her if I need anything. Tells me I should call my boyfriend. "He'll help you if you let him," she urges me. She doesn't want to see me go through this alone, but she knows me well. As soon as I hear the door close behind her, I pull the covers over my head and stay there for two days. I cannot watch movies because I don't have my best friend to pause and fast-forward. As I bleed through the last of the maxi pads, the list of places I cannot go swells: *grocery store, my favorite podcast, Instagram, dog park.*

When I finally let my boyfriend hold me, I am eight pounds lighter. My boyfriend takes me to the beach, and I add *beach* to the list of places I cannot go without being triggered. The post-abortion pamphlet says *most women are able to return to work and normal activities after a few days of rest.* I wait. My boyfriend waits. My dog waits. Everyone waits.

My friends start to recognize my depression. The check-in texts flow in, and I share about my abortion with a few select friends. I don't know what to say other than, "I was pregnant . . . and now I'm not." Everyone clocks the date—my abortion landing on the same day the Supreme Court overturned *Roe v. Wade*. Empathy swaddles the irony. Gratitude gets forced down my throat. *Can you imagine if . . . ?* I tell everyone that no, I cannot imagine. I don't tell them what I can imagine—what I can't stop myself from imagining—which is that if I could not have obtained an abortion that was safe, legal, and free, I would have gone to *any* lengths to end my pregnancy.

My friends ask me how I'm doing, *you know, with the emotional stuff?* Their confusion marches right up my grief, finger-wagging, and muses, *I thought you never wanted kids.* After this, I stop talking to my friends about my abortion and turn to my other best friend: Gin.

I spend the next several months trying desperately to numb and hide and outrun my grief. My grief confuses everyone, including me. I read the pamphlets again. I call the social worker. I take a leave from work. I wonder about the two women on either side of me in that abortion clinic and question if either of them is struggling like I am. Shame enters my life as Gin's wild cousin. Together, the three of us party. I lose my center.

***

Months later, I wake up in rehab and am forced to face my new friend Shame, without the soothing and numbing power of Gin. I start therapy and meet the impossible task of trying to describe why I feel so much crippling, gobsmacking, life-altering grief over losing something I never, ever wanted. My therapist brings me back to the moment I found out I was pregnant. I was alone, far from home, away from the very decent man I had decided to share my life with. I was gripping on to my eight months of sobriety. The day I found out I was pregnant, I was uncertain of so many things, but the one thing I was certain of was that I did not want to be a mother. All I had at that moment was my sobriety and my certainty. I booked my abortion almost immediately after seeing the positive test. I called my best friend first, my boyfriend a few days later. I asked her to come to the East Coast, asked him not to.

My therapist and I search for the conception of my grief in other places. The bathroom stall where I panicked and cried, where I took my first pregnancy test two weeks after I lost my virginity at fifteen. The friend I supported through a particularly devastating miscarriage last year. My own strained relationship with my mother. Finally, my therapist ushers me back to the abortion clinic and asks me to list every detail I could remember. "All I remember," I volunteer, "is waking up and asking the nurse, *where is the relief?*" My therapist delicately guides me through the memory with the help of my medical file. She reminds me that when I woke up, I was screaming, begging for the relief, and had to be restrained to the bed. She reminds me that I wept so hard I had to be admitted to the hospital. My therapist thinks I am experiencing PTSD and, like, the nurse from my hospital stay, reminds me that this is normal. While some women do feel relieved and "return to normal activities," many women have trauma and shame, and even regret. I curdle over the word "regret."

I have never wanted to be a mother. My parents joke that even when I was a child, I didn't enjoy being around other children. By the time I was a young adult, I vehemently proclaimed that I was not having children, even though I constantly faced the adage *you're young; you might change your mind.* I told all my partners that I was not interested in having children. I learned early that anyone who had the air of *you'll change your mind*—or, worse, *I'll change your mind*—was a major red flag and should be avoided. I was on birth control and always used protection, so the thought of ever getting pregnant lived far off in a distant land called My Worst Nightmare, but to be honest, I didn't think of it all that much.

In my early thirties, when most of my friends started becoming parents for the first time, I felt even more cemented in my choice. Being child-free allowed me the freedoms my friends craved, and I took advantage of those freedoms in any way I could—traveling solo, sleeping in, and being spontaneous, just to name a few. When the alarm bells of my biological clock started sounding and more people started asking me if kids were part of my plan, I was still certain that I did not want to be a mother.

"I have never wanted to be a mother or be pregnant or adopt a child or even be an aunt," I explain to my therapist. Her eyes indicate *but* . . . "But all I feel is grief." The grief in every cell that knows that I would likely never become a mother in the traditional sense of the word. The grief that was as swift and unsuspected as an earthquake the moment after I woke up from my abortion. The grief that I could not explain to anyone for months after my abortion. The grief that sticks to each key as I type this today.

***

Roe v. Wade was overturned on the same day my life went through the meat grinder. When it finally churned me out, I was a completely different animal. My therapist and I continue PTSD coping skills every week. My boyfriend and I have seen a grief counselor together, and I belong to an abortion support group. It has taken a whole team of people to help me return to work and normal activities. Every time Shame creeps in, I think of that nurse clutching my shoulder, reminding me this is all normal.

Leaving rehab just before Christmas, I feel safe enough to attend a small social gathering with three of my closest girlfriends. None of them have seen me in months, and I promise myself before I leave the house that I will not make this night about my grief. I will laugh and let myself feel the freedom that comes with being child-free and with ninety days of sobriety. Over a dark wood platter of olives, jammy fruit, and tangy cheese, my friends and I land in deep conversation, a place that feels comfortable and familiar. When the time feels right, I tell them about my abortion and, inevitably, I tell them about my grief. I wait for *but we thought you never wanted kids*. One friend takes my hand and says, "I felt the same way after mine." The other confesses that although she has two healthy children, she would consider it if she fell pregnant today. The third doesn't say anything but messages me the next day to tell me she is pregnant. That my grief is her mirror and that she hopes I hold on to it, find a way to nurture it. That I have something now that I didn't have before. Certainty. I plant that seed and watch it grow.

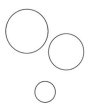

Anonymous Question Box for Eve

Deborah Meltvedt

Is masturbation a sin?

This is your first question of the day. You almost joke because it reminds you of one Family Life Committee meeting when a parent asserted that condoms and masturbation lead to the feminization of the military and the general downfall of America's youth. But you are well trained. Instead of saying *not a sin but a goddamn glory*, you say straight-faced to thirty-something tenth graders, *so, class, what do you think*?

I was a health sex educator. In public schools. I witnessed the struggle of reproductive truths rise and fall, then rise and fall again. I was careful navigating controversy and collective shame. To not bring my personal histories or political views through classroom doors. Often lauded with praise (*I could never do that!*), other times called a robber of morality and the giver of promiscuity. The snake in the garden luring Eve to Planned Parenthood.

I wish I were more honest to their questions in the classroom. That when I reached into the anonymous Sex Ed Question Box, I also pulled out my own truths buried in a world of secrets and shame.

Why do girls have periods?

Draw the uterus on the board. Keep yourself from turning the fallopian tubes into antlers on a moose. Focus on vocabulary—estrogen, follicles, ovulation. Don't let memory get in the way. Fifth-grade film, 1969. Disney one with Tinker Bell telling you the splendor of menstruation becomes the baby-making gift all women want. Remember being horrified. When blood comes two years later, you realize betrayal. Tinker Bell, as usual, had lied. No glory, just the embarrassment of pads fastened with straps that cut and loosened. Remember praying every day that boys would never notice.

C'mon, tell the class. Your body was the number thirty-two in gym class. Teachers, clipboards in hand, marked you absent if your white tennis-shoed feet were not covering your blacktop number. But five days each month, mortified, you said your number out loud. The sin of Eve was the words of menstruation. Out loud got you a private shower. Got you out of showing your nipples, butt, thighs, and pubic hair to forty-something peers and two matron gym teachers. At least in shame, private showers saved you from adolescent eyes watching your uterine lining flow down your legs.

What can I do for cramps?

You recite safety measures of warm baths, exercise, and maybe Advil (if Mom approves). Don't slip and say yours were so bad your doctor gave you Darvon. Opioids are covered in the alcohol and drug unit. This reminds you, a shot of whiskey also helps.

Why are your breasts so small?

I swear to god you will get this question. Well, maybe yours will be "Why are they so big?" or "Have you ever done it with a dog?" or "How old were you when you lost it?" Don't read it out loud; remind students *no personal questions please.* Yet you want to defend. Lecture how bras suck, and men have told you your boobs fit nicely into champagne glasses. So there.

But never take things personally.

Why is the dress code worse for girls?

Sigh. It's still true. Years ago, you loved those new velour hot pants, thinking you were one cool *Seventeen* magazine It Girl in homeroom. Till Shop Teacher called you out. Called you a whore via disguised lectures on what young ladies do and don't do while he stared at your legs swinging free. So you looked down, crossed your thighs, and learned you are the reason boys are out of control.

Inform your class, *as long you work hard, wear whatever the hell you want.*

What's an orgasm?

Hear a pin drop as you describe the physiology of thresholds. Avoid actually using the O-word at all possible costs. You are told this at the aforementioned Family Life meetings while judging six hours of puberty and reproduction films. You must catch your real words. If you don't, the boys and girls will spill onto each other and fuck each other between periods three and four. As if they've never watched HBO. Or porn sites.

Ideally you want to say "O" feels sometimes like a sneeze. Only a thousand times better.

What does cum taste like?

You will giggle. They like to *catch you* with a zinger. Breathe deep, shuffle feet, let thirty pairs of ears fall upon each dripping syllable, flush of cheekbones, and answer, *Well, some people report different experiences and blah blah blah.* In honesty, you want to kick every fringe member of any Family Life committee who thought sex ed needed to be tied up and scrubbed down. You want to tell these curious, horny kids something real—that it tastes like asparagus or sour milk, sometimes the last lick on a salt-rimmed margarita. Like the first juice Eve must have had in that wretched garden so long ago.

How bad is a pelvic exam?

Reveal you will never feel comfortable. Almost like dying each time they tell you to scoot down and relax with your bony butt against thin paper and your crotch open to the world. Good news, it won't take long. Good news, it can save your life. Learn to count tiles on the ceiling. To talk about anything—travel, sports, what you had for breakfast, while a stranger sticks their head between your legs.

Describe the clinic story. The one with the cute resident. Thick blond hair, deep blue eyes. Taking his turn in Reproductive Rotation. How you assisted holding out the instruments while smiling. The patient was only fifteen. First time in stirrups, shaking, cute resident between her thighs. She cannot help her muscled walls shut tight. His voice curt. *I can't do this if you don't relax.* Her eyes tearing. Her voice, soft, *I'm sorry, I'm sorry.* Gloves snap, him louder, *I'll be back when you learn to relax.*

You held her hand. Whispered, *No worries; it's not your fault.*

When it was over, the resident, not so cute anymore, asked you out. Your voice, loud: *Only when you learn not to be an ass.*

Hearing this, your class applauds. Together you sign imaginary pacts about speaking up for ourselves.

Do you have to be in love?

To marry or pick out patio furniture, to pay a mortgage, raise dogs and small children, yes, but not with sex. Think about the eight or twelve times you did it out of everything but love: lust, rebellion, curiosity, fear. Twenty thousand feet up because you thought the plane was going down and you drank too much and he unzipped your pants beneath the blanket that read Friendly Skies. Again, repeat, you thought you were going to die.

In reality, ask the class, *So, what do you think?*

Does birth control really work?

Recite Guttmacher Institute facts on birth control. Explain how far we've come. Make them think about the sacrifice of women. About your mother, desperate to take the Pill in clinical trials, but your physician Dad said no. When your little sister was born, your mom's fifth child in eight years, male doctors at St. Agnes Hospital denied her a tubal ligation. Tell students how your mother refused to hold Mary Kay meetings until they changed their minds.

You want to add your own stories. Inserting diaphragms that got stuck, or that made traveling with your boyfriend through New England a painful exercise of always having to pee. Describe the nauseous years of pills with a shitload of estrogen before experts realized one hundred micrograms was a bit too much. How now, after years of research on their moms' and grandmothers' hormones, the Pill is so much safer today.

So use it. Better yet, tell them to use condoms. Every time. The stakes are high.

What if he won't wear a condom?

Bypass if he loves you he will. Tell them flat out, boys/men will use them if you ask. Your first lover in college. Lawyers in sleazy motel rooms, your husband who never ever said no way. Rip open the package, wet your lips. Offer to put it on.

I know a friend who knows a friend whose (fill in the blank: boyfriend hits her. Stepfather touched her. Boyfriend raped her.).

In algebra, there are finite equations. Grammar has structure. DNA explains some meaning of life. But these questions are the read-between-the-lines muddy water lessons. You tell the class the first day you are a mandated reporter. So they tell you in code. You give back the usual: what is consent, who can help, and *it's not your fault.* You tell them to speak up, tell a counselor, their body is THEIR body. Inside of you, your heart shudders.

Isn't abortion murder?

If it's a boy asking, tell him he doesn't get to vote. If it's a girl, sigh deeply, say, *I really don't know.* Ask them to research. Each side. Sway them toward the ethics that a woman's life matters more. Be very, very careful.

Disclose that sometimes you drive by the downtown clinic to confront the protestors. To learn what they say. They wear sensible shoes and carry signs reading *Killers* and *All women regret.* You asked them once if they hand out condoms (you think like hate). The leader looked you up and down, twirled her sign like a cheerleader on the wrong but winning side, and said, *Those never work.*

Tell the kids they can have their beliefs, but they don't get to lie.

How come you never had children?

Your answer often changes. On soft days say you nurture by teaching. Other days you wanna make shit up. Talk long labors and a love for Saturday-morning Little League. Mostly you confess *it's complicated.* Maybe you can't. Maybe you just don't like the sound of babies screaming. Reassure them you love the sound of teenager curiosity.

Is masturbation a sin?

It comes up again. This time, admit not a sin but a gift. It's cheap, available, doesn't cause cancer or abortions. Learn to be as good as the French. They love cheese and wine and romance. Tell them the story of your first trip to Paris, where you watched a driver navigate traffic and the rhythm of his own penis coming to life in Parisian five o'clock traffic.

Tell them how you wanted to applaud.

Why is it hard being a girl?

Last question. Your mind makes a movie. You hear your mother singing you to sleep, then weeping at midnight. A boy snaps your bra strap in seventh grade. In college you wait three days for your first pregnancy test results, years later two weeks for HIV. You hold up signs with images of crossed-out coat hangers. A friend is raped. Best friends have abortions and later children they love. A trusted man forces you to *do this*. Your nieces march for a cause that once was then now is not. You vote. Three women a day are killed by someone once loved. You suffer marathons, not childbirth. Remember a lifetime of pads, tampons inserted, saying goodbye to uterine bleeding and hello to invisibility. You look for ways to look young. Explain to students it's Ms. not Mrs. or Miss. We all share personal pronouns. Six judges decide your great-nieces don't have rights to their own bodies. Teen pregnancy is down. Sexism up. ERA never ratifies. A condom breaks. Gender parties divide pink versus blue. Most women still take the man's last name. We look for love in right and wrong spaces.

How do you finally answer?

One girl speaks up. *It doesn't suck, but for some reason my body is scary as hell.*

Smiling, you think, *time to put away the box.* Give students the platform. One day one will co-teach contraception with their peers. Another will give a speech on menstrual equity. Many will march. New voices will rise. The good kind of out loud.

A gift perhaps, for Eve.

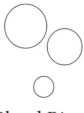

Blood Rites

Katey Funderburgh

My first blood comes in a snowstorm. I am fifteen, cheeks windburnt and red with cold, unwrapping a pad in the bathroom stall. Outside my small Colorado high school, ice has slicked over the sidewalk and snowdrifts reach up toward a whirling sky. The ends of my hair fall in front of my eyes as I look down, watch my blood drip hot and slow into the toilet. I try not to be afraid.

After school, I take the bus to my mother's work, pressing my forehead against the frosting windows to watch the storm shake more and more snow down before me. When my mom hugs me, I whisper it to her. She touches my cheek, says, *This is wonderful news, honey,* and tells me that we'll stop by the store later. She is already reaching into her pocket for her phone, already calling my grandmother.

I was raised in a house full of women: my mother, my grandmother, my younger sister, and me. When my hair grew long and unwieldy, my grandmother brought kitchen scissors out to the porch. I knelt beneath her as she cut. During one of these haircuts, she told me about our tradition: *When your mother got her period, I made her a cake.* She dragged a comb down my hair to measure out the uneven ends. *Chocolate with chocolate frosting. I didn't want her to be ashamed.* A drag of her cigarette. A series of snips. *We'll celebrate your first blood, too.* My mother has the same honey-colored hair as I do.

At the store with my mother, we select a tub of mint chocolate chip ice cream. My sister and grandmother are both at home, baking a Bundt cake. The sky is darkening; the moon is full and bright behind the storm clouds when my mom and I pull into the driveway. The snow from our clothes evaporates into the warm, sweet air of the kitchen. We eat the cake while it is still hot, and the ice cream melts into puddles on our plates. The storm makes our electricity flicker, so my sister lights candles in a cluster at the center of the table. My grandmother says that it is like a first birthday—the first day that I am able to make another life inside me, christened by the women in my family. Their faces glint in the candlelight.

I keep trying not to be afraid. All I know of womanhood begins with the sacrifices that I watched my mother and grandmother make for me and my sister, for the protection of their own bodies. I place my palm low on my belly, over my jeans, where I think my uterus sits. I'm not a child anymore—I am a bleeding body capable of motherhood, and I'm so afraid that I won't be good enough for it. This is my inheritance—my sudden consciousness of all I will have to bear to become someone brave, someone worth loving. Someone like them.

At age twenty, my grandmother moved alone to San Francisco to work in the heart of the women's rights movement. She rented out a studio apartment for herself and her pet rat, cheekily named Rat-Rat. She set up an easel in one corner, her bed in the other, and placed Rat-Rat on top of her dresser, where she could overlook the fire escape whenever my grandmother was out. Sometimes

Rat-Rat would escape her cage and gather my grandma's jewelry and cigarette butts in her mouth. She stashed these all around the apartment: inside pillowcases, in between couch cushions, under the fridge, in the little divots of crusted paint palettes that my grandmother left scattered around.

Then one night, the man came. He was a vengeful lover, or a complete stranger, or a friend she'd turned down once or twice—this part of her story changed each time it was retold, like oil shimmering on a puddle's surface. He crawled up the fire escape and forced the window open. Rat-Rat started to scream. My grandma woke to the man standing above her, knife in one hand, undoing his belt buckle with the other. Rat-Rat's little hands shook the bars of her cage, and she kept screaming, louder and louder. The man dropped his knife and ran.

My girl saved me, she tells me when I am twelve and sitting criss-cross at her feet. She dangles her cigarette in the side of her mouth while her fingers, swelling with arthritis, slowly weave my hair into braids. *I was in San Fran to protect women, and my girl Rat-Rat was protecting me!* She laughs, my hair in her hands. I wish I could turn around and check her eyes for signs of fear. She blows smoke around me like a shawl, then continues. *There were all the marches, and getting women to vote. There were meetings every night. And the day that* Roe v. Wade *passed! How proud we felt.* There is sunlight slanting across the porch boards, casting shadows on my lap.

I try not to be afraid. But when I am nineteen, I am in bed with a boy, and I feel like glass. I cannot tell if I am opening for him, or if he can see through me. Blood falls like rain in the wind onto my sheets.

Mid-January gets dark at 6:30 p.m. in Colorado. The cold is the kind that leaks into my bone marrow. The snowflakes that freeze on the windowpane of my dorm room are perfect and clear. I can see each one, can move the tip of my index finger from one small flake to the next. A halo of fog blooms on the glass around the tip of my finger. I am wrapped in a blanket, shaking slightly, while the boy is down the hall taking a piss. He is freckled and angry most of the time, gentlest when he is moving his hands down my spine. I want to be loved, so I take it.

 The first girl knocks on my door in April. She is crying softly, saying, *Sorry, sorry, I didn't know.* Then the second girl. *None of us knew he was dating you.* Then the third. Then the fourth, and then I stop counting. I let each girl inside my room, and she sits on my bed. After each confession, I say *Thank you* and *I'm not mad.* My fear opens its heavy eyes, spreads through my body, and settles into anger like mounds of perfect snow. I bear it until I can't, until I am screaming at the boy in a parking lot. He says nothing except *Fuck you* over and over again, and I am afraid of the shame that tucks itself behind my rising voice.

My mother was born gentle. We are in the kitchen washing shorn branches from a raspberry bush when she tells me that her first memory is of a mother cat giving birth to a litter of kittens in her crib. She hands me a branch and I notice that the birthmark on her left wrist matches mine. It is spring, and I am seventeen. I had woken up that morning with a fever and nausea from cramps. My mother placed her hand on my cheek, then ran her finger along the spines of her books and pulled out the ones on herbal medicine. She held each up to my grandmother. *Is it this one? Or this?* And when my grandmother nodded, listed the page number by heart, my mother showed me the list of herbal remedies for period pain. We set off into the forest behind our house, our breath making little clouds in the icy morning air.

 I kept the kittens a secret all night, my mother recalls, *and I loved them so completely.* She moves intuitively, pulling each leaf from its stalk and gathering them into a bundle. She sets a pot to boil and directs me to the couch, tucking me in with a blanket. *But not as much as I love you!* A kiss on the top of my head.

When my mother left my father, she buckled my sister and I into our car seats and drove all night to her mother's doorstep. She didn't want to—couldn't—raise us alone, and my grandmother wouldn't let her.

The tea is warm, and my mother is steadfast. All the difficult world, and still her womanhood is built on a love so big I'm afraid that I will fail it. My fever breaks and the fear pulses through me.

The winter I turn twenty-one, I do not bleed at all. There is an infection that crawls inside my uterus and makes me cramp, but no blood comes. Past sunset in early February, I walk alone to Safeway. Each of my steps lands on dirty, crusted snow. I think about the doctor I begged to help me last month, standing in my paper gown, feeling like I did when I was small and gripping my mom when she kissed me goodnight, afraid that if she left, someone would kidnap me in the middle of the night. This fear of terrors I cannot see, driving me to urgent care when the pressure inside my uterus grew and grew. *It's just a yeast infection*, the doctor smiled at me. *Go home and rest, okay?*

At Safeway, I purchase just a bottle of champagne and a tube of over-the-counter yeast infection medication. I know already that my body won't respond to it, that if the last tube didn't help, this one won't, either. But I cannot recall any of the names of my mother's herbs, and I don't know how to tell her how this has happened to me.

He wasn't always violent. I had loved him, actually. This man I was dating—*twenty-one is too young for marriage*, I had said, *and I can't stay with you if that's what you want from me*. The relationship ended quietly.

There had been small signs—the way he was jealous of my friends, how his grip tightened just a bit too hard when I'd leave his house, the lies I told to keep him from meeting my family—and as I pop the cork of my champagne in the dark on my walk home, I wish I'd seen it coming sooner. The infection feels like it's my fault. I place my hand low on my belly, take a swig of champagne. *I'm sorry*, I think, *I didn't mean to hurt you*. I think about Rat-Rat, about the kittens. Have I failed? Good women are gentle. Good women know better. Good women aren't scared.

The breakup breaks something in this man I loved. There are shadows of him around bends in the sidewalk. He screams at me across campus, leaves letters under my door, and emails me with detailed lists of everything that is wrong with me, and everything he'll do to me if I don't change my mind and take him back. Something about this violence feels predictable. I am trying to bear it. I am trying to prove that I am a good woman.

Tipsy from the champagne, I stomp snow off my boots in the entrance of my home and hear my friends calling from the kitchen to tell me dinner is ready. Their circle has tightened around me all winter. They let me sleep in their beds. One of them walks with me to campus, and another walks me home. My mailbox fills with their letters, so that his becomes just another envelope of many that I open each day. In my shame, in the pain I am holding in my uterus, my friends are patient and protective.

At home, I hold up the tube of medication like a trophy, then sit down to a plate of mac and cheese. *You should know*, one of them says to me, *he's starting to message us too*.

All their faces at the table. All of my fear.

I remember my sister's hands lighting the candles when I was fifteen.

The next morning, I file the restraining order. I am aching and afraid in the Title IV office at my school, watching snow blow silently past the office windows. I float just above my body and repeat like an incantation in my head: *I cannot let this fear be theirs, I cannot let this fear be theirs.*

I hold my breath until there are small yellow heads of spring flowers popping up along the edges of the sidewalk. Springtime, and no one has heard from the man at all. My infection trickles slowly toward healing. Slowly, I let myself exhale, feeling all the knots of my fear fall away. All I had made myself bear in the name of womanhood dissipates like sand falling through your hand. Like rain steaming on the concrete. Like knowing that the women who saved you are safe too.

Love is not a test. We do not survive alone.

It is spring, and I am lying in the grass, one hand thrown over my eyes to keep out the sun, and I feel it: blood, hot and sudden.

I go inside and unwrap a pad in the bathroom. My hair falls in front of my eyes. This ritual, this marker of my womanhood, this blood that the women who raised me carried in them too—it had been gone from me for so long, I had forgotten how to love it.

On the cusp of the autumn I turn twenty-four, my grandmother dies. It is 1 a.m. in late September. The air smells like it might snow soon, and the aspens are beginning to yellow. My sister slips the rings off our grandmother's fingers and places one on our mother's hand, one on mine, and one on her own. Then we all reach out to each other and form a circle above her dying body. I want her to take a last gulping breath, to cry out, to say something, but instead her eyes are closed, and she dies in a way that I cannot hear. But I feel her, like a hot slow wind, drifting gently upward.

I do not feel afraid. I sleep in my mother's bed with her, and when the morning breaks, I get up and begin to bake a cake.

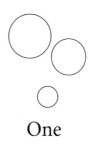

One

Katie Clausen

3

Adhering posters to a ceiling must be a tough job. Pushing thumbtacks into perforated drywall tiles while standing atop a ladder would mess with my depth perception. Why didn't they use Command strips? If sharp pins landed on a pregnant lady on this exam table, there would be lawsuits. I'd have to find a new IVF clinic.

I'm not a pregnant lady. The ceiling poster reminds me of that. It screams 1992, with its depiction of bleached green ovaries like martini olives and Starburst-pink fallopian tubes. There are other organs I memorized in high school biology and promptly forgot. Muscles. Bones. Ligaments.

Fetus. Hugging itself.

I guess the female reproductive cycle doesn't change much. No need for a new poster.

A clammy palm settles on my thigh. "Ready for the ultrasound?"

The nurse's lipstick is stop-sign red. For some reason, when she pulls my legs apart, my mind leaps to an image of Moses parting the Red Sea.

"I'm inserting the wand."

I glue my eyes to the poster.

It's impossible not to gasp when a cold, carrot-shaped probe is shoved up into the softest place inside. My thighs seize as the nurse presses down on my abdomen. Grayscale images rise on the computer monitor on a medical cart beside me. I can't decide if my insides look like a plate of sushi rolls or the tangled knitting project I abandoned last month. Circles adjust in size as the nurse guides the probe around.

She points to the center of the screen. Wrist hairs poke out from the edge of her tight disposable gloves. "A few follicles are eighteens."

Eighteen millimeters. I'm starting to understand the fertility jargon.

"They need more development."

Development. As if I'm a marketing campaign for a seasonal flavor of Cheerios.

I let out a quick breath. "How many days before surgery?"

She rolls her chair away from the exam table. "Hard to predict. The doctor will decide when you'll get the trigger shot."

"You saw them. What do you think?"

"Hmmm," she half sings, half coughs.

They're always lullabying around here, harmonizing with the baby photos on the walls.

When I sit up, the snap-crackle-pop of the white medical paper crinkles underneath me. "Do they look healthy?"

"The doctor will update you tomorrow. You're shivering. Please get dressed."

I waddle over and plop down on the doctor's stool, my stomach bloated and the skin around my belly button raw from hormone injections. As I wipe sweat from my brow, my eyes wander to a chart above the sink. Embryonic Development. The mechanical words march in my brain, typewriter-like. *Human embryogenesis. Fertilization. Oocyte.*

Oocyte. A cell. An almost-egg.

I close my eyes. I have oocytes. They are mine. Finally, a part of my body that's all mine.

2

"Did you know your thyroid is malfunctioning?"

The doctor sits spine-straight behind her desk. She is thin-boned with a kind half smile and capillaries prominent behind her eyes. I draw imaginary lines between the tiny blood vessels, an internal game of connect the dots.

I suppress a shudder. "No."

She leans in, hands folded. "You're underweight."

I drop my lower lip, pretending to be surprised.

"Are you tired frequently?"

"Yes."

"Cold?"

I nod.

"Dry skin?"

I close my eyes. "Will this affect the surgery?"

"You'll need medication immediately after it," she says. "Autoimmune conditions complicate fertility. Your thyroid must be under control before we fertilize."

"I'm not fertilizing."

She raises her eyebrows. "What?"

"I'm freezing them."

She reclines in her chair and bites down on a pen. "At age thirty-five, fertility declines."

"I'm aware."

"You're financially stable," she says. "You're a beauty. Motherhood would suit you."

The edges of the chair sharpen against my hips. "I guess motherhood is divulged only to those of its own favorited company."

"You're a poet too."

I want to push in her nose, a Pinocchio in reverse.

"Any history of thyroid problems in the family? Hashimoto's disease, thyroiditis iodine deficiency?"

I shake my head.

"Radiation therapy?"

"No."

"Anorexia?"

My breath catches. "Anorexia," I repeat. I don't have to nod. She sees the yes in my eyes.

"Did you ever lose your menstrual cycle?"

I half wince, half nod.

She leans back in her chair. "Do you think your body could carry a child?"

The muscles in my neck tighten like a wind-up toy. "Wouldn't you know that more than me?"

"What I mean is, could you feed yourself enough consistent nutrition?"

There's something in her gaze I can't point to. Compassion? No. Impatience? Maybe.

"Restriction could be fatal for the baby," she says. "Your body would be someone else's."

A scoff escapes my lips. Nothing I'm not used to.

She gives me a long, level look. "Was that a laugh?"

My voice stumbles. "No."

Her eyebrows scrunch like inchworms. "Anorexia is a protection. A hiding."

I search the ceiling for a poster. "I'm not hiding."

"Perhaps there's some unprocessed trauma?"

I think about walking out, but my legs are rubber bands. I want to take twenty steps past this moment.

She looks out the window. Right then, I recognize the look. Pity.

"Eating disorders cause significant wear and tear."

Wear and tear. Like I'm a book tossed between schoolchildren.

She reaches across her desk and cups her hand over mine. "You don't have to do this alone."

"Do what?"

"IVF. Life."

She doesn't know.

I want to do it alone.

1

"Guess what, sweetheart?" The nurse's lipstick is a soft nude today, a layer of gloss reflecting the fluorescent ultrasound light.

She presses down on my abdomen and guides the probe near my cervix. At this point, the machine feels like a third limb.

"I think tomorrow's the day."

I sit up halfway. "Really?"

"You have some twenties."

The screen radiates. Oocytes glow. Round and distended bubbles. Like little planets.

"Did you always want to be a mom?"

A hot tingle zips up my spine. It's the first time I've heard the word "mom" in reference to myself.

I used to equate motherhood with the pressure of stocking the family with grandchildren. The thought of taking care of another person felt like squishing myself into the small end of a tunnel. But there's always been a deep-tissue longing. A hoping that inched toward knowing. Protecting and guiding someone—the right someone—for once. Witnessing the unfolding of someone's story. Knowing what unyielding love is like.

"Yes," I say, unwaveringly. "I did."

The doctor enters the exam room. Her maroon sweater with snowflakes and reindeer silhouettes makes her seem more human. The air in the room stiffens. The look on her face feels disguised; soft ballerina tulle wrapped around needles. Like she thinks I've grown into the wrong kind of woman.

My tongue is heavy inside my mouth. It weighs almost as much as my heart.

Our eyes meet, and she gives me a top-shelf smile. "Six a.m. tomorrow. We're on."

0

The surgery is twenty-three minutes long. After, my insides feel scraped out like a jack-o'-lantern.

At home, I can't sleep. The taste of anesthesia, like cold ash, sits on the top layer of my tongue. Just as I'm drifting off, my phone buzzes. The hospital. I gasp for air and answer it.

"How many?"

The doctor clears her throat. "One successful oocyte was retrieved."

I don't have spit to swallow. "One?"

"That's correct."

My fingers go numb. "Why . . . ?"

"I wish I had better news," she says. "It's unpredictable."

One?

"There are options moving forward."

"Like another $19,000?"

"Another cycle would—"

I throw the phone against the wall.

One.

My brain erupts. Starts to tell the stories. *Don't eat.* This is my fault. *Don't move.* My body's fault. *If you don't move, it will all stop soon.* My body tenses. *Move. Run off all that extra flesh, the almost-hips.*

I burst out of bed, push my feet into my boots, and plunge out the door. It's two degrees outside. I don't have a hat or mittens, but I don't feel cold.

Injections. Bloating. Probes shoved up inside me every two days. Hormones, bleeding, fainting.

I run.

The flash of an image. My knees pried apart.

Run.

Another flash. A monstrous body hovering above me.

"One . . . " I speak out loud, harsh wind burning my cheeks.

Tears well behind my eyes. I push them back in with my fingertips.

Pressing. Moving inside me. Pain.

I run, the same word escaping my lips.

One.

My boots are losing their tread. My heart is losing its tread.

Unremember. The hunger on his face.

Unremember. That night. The ER. The nurse's quivering voice as she inserted the speculum. *Honey, you're torn apart in there.*

Unremember. The STD injections. The gigantic pill. *To prevent pregnancy.*

One.

One night. Torn apart.

My knees give out. I collapse onto the boulevard, machine-like. Face first into the snow. My arms won't lift. My fingers won't move.

It hurts.

I'm feeling.

My toes tingle.

I'm feeling.

This isn't about hormones. It's not about bleeding or bloating.

One after another, the tears come. Then I'm heaving, retching. Droplets turn into salt on my cheeks.

This is about anger. My twenties could have its own twenty-two-episode Netflix series, each one featuring a time a man touched my body when I didn't want him to, where I didn't want him to.

This is about fear. I cringe when someone touches my back out of nowhere. I don't know what it's like to sleep through the night. While women casually peel off their swimsuits in the gym locker room, I drape a towel over my body and wait for an empty stall before slowly inching my suit down, hiding even from myself. Spreading my knees apart in yoga poses catapults me back to places I want to unremember. Sex feels like a contract I never signed but still abide by.

This is about shame. A secret that causes me to keep the doors unlocked at night, tempting the universe to give up on me. For all the nights and all the men after. The very animal of my body—marrow, sinews, veins—was something stripped and consumed. I half waited, half wanted the next someone to groom me and take me for a ride. Put me back in the 12x12 stall when they're done, where I'd be unable to move until the next one came.

This is about hunger. A desperation, a craving for intimacy, but being unable to tolerate it. For my life to be more than far-flung dots, meaningless and unconnected.

So I turned the sword on myself. Cut the fat off my body. Unwelcome weight. The memory of unwanted hands on me.

I erased it all.

After

There is one egg in a freezer somewhere in Illinois. My own little possibility.

I try to keep my finger on the pulse of now. Half hope, half reality. At thirty-eight, I'm considered high-risk. Even if I did get pregnant, the things that could go wrong are as long as a Thanksgiving grocery list. There's ripe sadness that my body may never hold life.

But what if it could?

At my follow-up appointment after surgery, I'm paying my bill at the clinic. Two women, one wearing an olive-green bomber jacket and the other a rainbow-striped dress covering a gigantic baby bump, are checking out. One woman wraps her arm around the other's shoulder.

A nurse calls out a name. The woman in rainbow stripes waddles over.

"Say hi to the *Saved by the Bell* poster for me," says the woman in the jacket.

I chuckle. "The ceiling poster from the nineties?"

The woman turns toward me and beams. "It's so raunchy, right? I make fun of it constantly. Gotta have humor when you're going through this for a year."

"A year?"

She nods. "It took three cycles for us. You?"

"I just froze my eggs," I say. "Well, egg."

"What do you mean?"

I let out a deep exhale. It reaches the tips of my toes. "I got one egg."

The woman's shoulders energize, and her eyes bloom. "All you need is one."

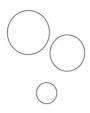

A Story of Two Births

Jennifer Alessi

After three years of fertility injections, I didn't want any pain. I'd attended childbirth classes, glossing over the breathing techniques, focusing on the epidural. My OB, a petite, no-nonsense New York City transplant, eschewed elaborate birth plans, especially at my "advanced maternal age." She endorsed the epidural. Beyond its sanctioned numbness, my husband and I joked, "The only plan is Dr. Chan."

She determined I should be induced on my due date. Kiera was fully formed, and my blood pressure risky. For the past month, per Dr. Chan's orders, I'd stopped daily at a drugstore to check my blood pressure on its public machine. Laying my arm in its cuff, I'd fret: *What if, during labor, a blood clot congealed and launched?* It didn't escape me that roughly seven hundred women in the United States die from maternity complications each year.

I was to report to the hospital at 5 p.m. Until then, I spent the day with my mother. We drove to Target for an air mattress should she and my husband both want to sleep in the room. I didn't trust my feet on the escalator (how many women had miscarried, tumbling from one?), so we took the elevator instead. The twin mattress was cheap, a fraction of the king and queen.

Beaming, we headed to a register, where the cashier and item scan confirmed the price was actually forty dollars more.

"But the shelf says $19.99." My bulging stomach had been an advantage for months.

Not with her.

"No," she stated, "it doesn't."

"It does."

"Why don't we check?" my mother suggested, squeezing my hand.

The cashier flicked off her register light. "Let's go."

"And if the shelf says $19.99, I get it for that?"

"It doesn't."

Magnanimous, a soon-to-be mother, I added, "But if the shelf says $59.99, I'll pay it."

I gloated over the luck of this discount.

But after a lunch out (my last meal for a while), when we got to the hospital in Glendale, it was deemed that we couldn't use the air mattress after all. Self-inflating, it could overload an outlet. I'd called and asked permission, but I didn't argue. Vitals taken, strapped into a gown, I reclined in a hospital bed. My husband arrived, and the mood turned festive. Giddy, my mother fished tiny wine bottles from her purse. She handed one to my husband while I feigned disapproval. A few remote clicks and I found *Grey's Anatomy*. What was Meredith up to? What marvel was she performing while being pursued by which intern? It felt indulgent just to lounge. My first trimester, Dr. Chan had warned—because of my age and blood pressure—she might put me on bed rest. Secretly, I was pleased. No more teaching and grading; I'd binge-watch *The Good Wife* and *Scandal*. That never happened, but this would do.

Then a nurse arrived to induce me. I'd been through countless pelvic exams, prided myself on not complaining. Most recently, Dr. Chan had clicked into the room, high heels and Louis Vuitton purse, patting my knee before leaving.

This nurse thrust a hand up inside me.

"Wider," she prodded. "Don't clench."

Frowning, she twisted her hand—bruising an organ? Wincing, I gripped the bed rails, desperate not to squirm. *Something's not right*, I nearly cried.

But then, she was done. Tablets inserted, she withdrew her arm.

I felt my insides uncoiling back into place.

Peeling off her gloves, she counseled, "It might take a while."

"I'll want an epidural."

She smiled before leaving. "Just push the call button."

In no time, the room began to tilt. One moment, the glint of clinking Sutter Home, the next, the TV undulating.

"Turn it off," I whimpered.

One or both leaned in. "What, honey?"

"Turn that fucking shit off."

Someone hit the call button. No one came. Someone rushed to the nurses' station; still no one came. The contractions, a creature, twisted my uterus, lancing with its nails. I tried to breathe through them, but there was no space, no time.

"Epidural! Epidural!"

My pleas died in the corridor's stillness. An intercom cracked to life: *All available . . . report to . . .* White coats, stethoscopes flapping against breasts, flew down the hall, followed by a hush that felt like fear.

Eventually, a different nurse appeared, checked my vitals and dilation, then sat down beside me and took my hand. "We haven't forgotten about you. We're updating Dr. Chan."

"I need an epidural. The pain is too much."

She wiped a cloth across my brow. "Of course." Her voice turned tight, hesitant. "There's an emergency down the hall—a woman in labor. All doctors are needed there. It'll just be a while."

A while lasted four hours.

Alongside the pain was the knowledge that another woman who'd had her last meal, her expectant day, was in trouble. I sensed there was something seriously wrong. Huddled, desperate voices ruffled the silence.

The anesthesiologist arrived—sitting me up, baring my back. And alongside the numbness (a liquid, pooling warmth), I understood, somehow, that the other mother was gone.

When the nurse returned, chin trembling, I said, "She didn't make it?"

"No."

"What happened?"

"I shouldn't say."

"Please."

She glanced into the hallway then near tears answered, "An embolism. Out of nowhere."

"Was she alone?" I needed to know that she hadn't been alone.

"Her husband was there."

I nodded. It mattered. And yet it didn't matter at all.

Another check and then Dr. Chan stroked my arm. "You're not dilated enough. And your baby's cord is wrapped around her neck. The safest course at this point is a C-section."

I cried then. "Anything."

Down the hall, in the operating room, she drew a curtain across my waist to block the cutting. The anesthesiologist kindly slipped the oxygen mask toward my cheek when I'd begged him to let me breathe. Soon, I heard my daughter's shrieking wail and the *ding! ding!* of a monitor celebrating time of birth. Her wobbly father cut the cord, then laid her in my arms. As I gazed and cooed, I commanded myself, "Never forget how lucky you are."

And for the five years since—pushing Kiera on a swing, comforting her when she cries, helping her complete a jigsaw puzzle—I haven't forgotten. But I don't think that's of any consequence to the woman down the hall, or her husband. Nor does it matter that my great-grandmother died in childbirth, leaving three kids to orphanages, her last words, *Oh, my poor children!* The woman down the hall rages. She roars, "How dare you?" She admonishes, "You know nothing."

So why write about it?

Because her story occurred next to mine. I can't write about my birth story without acknowledging her death.

I imagine the white sheet cloaking her deathbed. I see myself tucking a blue sheet around Kiera's legs, and a faceless woman draping a yellow blanket around her son's narrow shoulders. A love so fierce must be eternal.

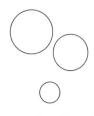

Into the Dark

Stephanie Vessely

The morning after Christmas, I come downstairs and see my keys hanging from the light switch nearest the garage door—instead of on their usual hook on the adjacent wall. Twenty years ago, I would have looked at the keys and thought, *yikes, I drank too much. I shouldn't have driven home last night.* But I am over five years sober at this point. I text a picture to my closest friend with a message about the spirit of perimenopause. I am turning forty-five the next day, and, it suddenly seems, fully on the journey.

The symptoms have trickled in slowly for the last several years. Like a roller coaster slowly ticking upward, I've known my time is coming. It started with a hot flash here, a hot flash there. Some unexplained rage. Migraines when I ovulate and when I menstruate. But in the last six months or so, things have really picked up. My anxiety is off the charts. I get teary on the regular. My period, normally so predictable I know its arrival to the day, has begun fluctuating between short and long cycles—but only sometimes. My heart palpitates. I am regularly haunted by a vague sense of existential dread. I can't seem to use enough lotion—my whole body is dry, dry, dry. I wake up in the middle of the night drenched in sweat. My ponytail is decidedly thinner. It also hurts my scalp to wear a ponytail. Is this a symptom of perimenopause? I don't know. It's just another in the long list of the ways my body is suddenly foreign to me.

I've been trying to prepare the best I can for whatever is coming. I've been reading books, the internet, whatever I can find. I am desperate for any semblance of knowing or control in the matter. What I keep finding instead: an undefined black hole; silence, but also a lot of conflicting voices; many, many shrugs. After all this time, here in the 2020s, the era in which my childhood promised there would be flying cars and time travel and robots who waited on us, it seems that what happens to a woman for anywhere from five to fifteen years in the middle of her life is still a vast mystery.

Other women I've asked don't shed much light. My mother insists she does not remember much about her transition into menopause, but my aunts tell me that she had intense mood swings, anxiety, depression. My closest friend, who is a couple of years younger than me, has been suffering the worst of early-onset menopause for years now. Others I've asked—friends who are older than me—haven't noticed any symptoms at all. I've read memoirs of women for whom it is the worst of times; others for whom it is, well, not the best of times, but not so terrible, either. The experience seems to vary wildly, with no rhyme or reason, no timeline, no set beginning or end. For me—a planner, a hyper-organized control freak—this is not welcome news.

I feel like I should have something profound to say about the coming loss of my period. Or like I should be looking forward to a life free from dealing with it all: the cramps, the bloating, making sure I always have tampons with me, just in case. Mostly, I feel like I'm on the precipice of something big, and I have no idea what it's going to be like. Like I'm about to get on a ride at an amusement park, but I don't know if it's the aforementioned roller coaster or a Tilt-A-Whirl or a float down the lazy river.

Based on observation, it seems like I'm supposed to go through this really big thing pretty quietly and mostly alone. That I'm supposed to, like the last thirty years of menstruating, hide that anything is happening at all. Just like I've gone to school and work and exercised and cooked and cleaned and socialized and done caretaking while sometimes bleeding, sometimes bleeding heavily, while sometimes suffering from a migraine, while sometimes feeling so very anxious that I want to crawl out of my skin, while sometimes almost doubled over with cramps, while sometimes so tired I can barely hold a conversation, I'm supposed carry on for the next however many years as if my body does not have needs or expectations. As if my body does not exist.

The thing about amusement park rides is that there are precautions in place. The operators make sure you're tall enough. They go over the safety information before the ride begins. They demonstrate how to wear the seat belt properly and make sure you are strapped in before the ride. With menopause, perimenopause, there are no operators. I'm seemingly in charge of everything—starting and stopping the ride, making sure I don't fall out—but no one has told me anything about how the ride works.

I do feel sad about my period ending. Or I feel sad about the things I've learned recently about menstruation—things I should have known all along. I didn't know until a few years ago, for instance, that my cycle has phases, and that each one comes with its own energy levels. Maybe if I had known, I could have planned my weeks and days accordingly. Maybe my menstruating years could have been less challenging, less chaotic.

I also wonder what the last thirty years would have been like if I were allowed to experience my period as something I didn't need to hide or be ashamed of. If the discourse weren't relegated to boyfriends pointing out when I was acting "crazy," or I didn't overhear remarks about being hormonal. What if someone had told me that my intuition is super strong right before and during my period? What if my fifth-grade health class had a unit on listening to our bodies, the messages contained in our cycles, the ways we can harness the power of our periods instead of, like the pads and tampons we stuffed in our bras and up our sleeves, pretending it wasn't there?

I've been thinking lately of my first period. Of that morning when I took my rust-stained underwear to my mother, who was getting ready in her bathroom, and asked her if she thought it was my period. I remember the confusion of it. I had been expecting my first period to be like the locker room scene in *Carrie*—gushing, dripping, bright red blood that needed to be, as the other girls screamed, plugged up. But this was much quieter. There was no gushing of anything. It wasn't even red. My mother studied my underwear but wasn't 100 percent sure, either. She thought it likely was my period and told me to wear a pad for the day and see what happened.

I remember the thrill of telling my friends that I, too, was now part of the club. But a club implies a knowing, a secret knowledge that those on the outside don't have. And we did have that—we finally had direct experience of what we had learned in the unit on our changing bodies that spring. But there was so much we didn't know and never would—why some of us had excruciating cramps and some of us had none at all. Why some of our periods lasted four days and others' periods lasted eight or nine. Why sometimes we skipped a period, even though we were all virgins. Menstruation, it seemed, was also entrance into the club of *not* knowing. Of waiting to see what happens. Of bringing bodily happenings and maladies to friends and doctors and rarely getting a certain answer. Perimenopause seems to be more of the same.

But I do not want it to be. I want to know how to make the most of this time. I want the culture to acknowledge that it's happening. I want to be able to call work and say *Hi, my brain is full of fog, so I'm going to work from home today*. Or better yet, *I'm not going to work today at all*. I want others to know that, as in puberty, my moods, emotions, and energy levels are in constant flux. That I am at times reactionary, or unable to function at peak ability. That sometimes I feel like I have been taken over by body snatchers. That I am doing the best I can. I would like some grace.

I am asking a lot, I know. I am asking for a reordering of society. For offices and schools and churches and communities to change how we operate. I am asking for our culture to be oriented toward something other than consumption, the economy, dollar bills. For our value to be tied to something other than the bottom line and how well we pretend not to have limitations and needs. I do not want to spend the next five to ten years pretending that what is happening to me isn't happening. I do not want to hide my hot flashes or my emotions. I want to be present for everything going on in my body—without shame, or embarrassment, or fear.

In junior high and high school, my friends and I called our periods Aunt Edna. We said we were on the rag or that it was that time of the month. The euphemisms are endless—the red tide, the monthly visitor, shark week, crimson tide, the curse, moon cycle, Aunt Flo.

I never thought to question these euphemisms back then, how they separate us from menstruation, how they hide it. It was just the way things were. I knew inherently that my period was something we didn't talk about with just anybody. But I also knew that it was kind of an afterthought—a thing going on in the background of my real life that should mostly be ignored, or at the very least, quietly tolerated. No one factored in whether someone had intense cramps while they were supposed to be taking a test, or whether an outburst of emotion might have a truth to it that shouldn't be dismissed just because they had their period.

In a world where women and girls are bombarded with marketing that implores us to guard against "embarrassing" leaks, that insist that "that time of the month" need not be different than other weeks—that we can still swim and play tennis (in white skirts) and generally carry on as if nothing is happening—where visual depictions of menstrual fluid are inexplicably blue, where no one ever needs to think we are feeling anything other than fantastic, it makes sense that the culmination of it all would be more hiding, more separating, more pretending the thing isn't the thing. That we would have a new euphemism—The Change.

It doesn't feel like a euphemism, though—it feels like an actual change is about to occur. Armed with information or not, the one thing I know for sure is there is nothing to be done about it. The only way around, as they say, is through. Maybe I cannot find answers because there are no answers to be found. There is no control to be had.

Perhaps the amusement park ride that is the most apt metaphor is the Old Mill ride from when I was a kid, where you float on a device of some kind—in my case a boat made to look like a hollowed-out log—into the dark tunnel for a while. Some versions were called the Tunnel of Love, and were romantic, relaxing, encouraging couples to cuddle. At my childhood amusement park, the path through the waters was dark, winding, shadowy, with sounds and animatronics designed to startle you. I rode that ride enough times to no longer be afraid—I knew where things were going to jump out and where I would hear screams. But the tunnel I'm about to enter remains a mystery. I will go anyway, because it's too late to stop the ride—and they won't let me get off even if I try. The only thing I can do is enter the fray. The only thing I can do is get to the other side.

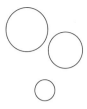

Self-Defense Posture

Monica Prince

In 2020, I asked my gynecologist for sterilization. I was thirty, madly in love with a polyamorous Black man named Rob, and settling into my tenure-track professorship at Susquehanna University. I still felt invincible the way young people do when their responsibilities are annoying but not difficult—laundry, bills, feeding oneself. The one thing I knew for sure: I didn't want to have biological children.

There was a long period in my life where I expected to get married and have children before I turned thirty; say, from infancy until 2012. That's what people do, right? They get an education, find a suitable lover, get a job, get married, buy a house, have kids, retire, die. A simple order that many of us have followed for a few millennia now to ensure the continuation of our species. Seems to work for most folks.

When my father got married for the fourth time in 2013, I started to believe that maybe this life trajectory wasn't quite what I wanted. Sure, I got educated, found several lovers, and hoped for a job once I graduated with my MFA in 2015. But the marriage and babies thing started to feel like a dress that fit six months ago and technically fits now that you've lost thirty pounds, but it flatters you less and you can't stop messing with it during meetings.

Verbose, yes. Nonetheless accurate.

By the time I moved to Selinsgrove, Pennsylvania, in 2017, I decided I didn't want kids. Newly polyamorous and still reckless with my body, I resigned myself to adoption. If I ever became stable enough to care for another human being, of course.

I sat across from my doctor. My current birth control method was expiring at the end of the year, and I didn't want to re-up. I needed to get these tubes tied now.

***

At two in the morning one night, a lover asked when I knew I didn't want kids.

I remember the moment vividly. 2017. Elwin, the love of my life for two years and change, was sitting in traffic with me, in the passenger seat of my Nissan Maxima, explaining what life he'd planned for himself once he'd paid off his student loans. He described the commune he'd build, a place all his lovers and their lovers could live and raise children together. He painted a (frankly super hippie-sounding) life of co-parenting, orgies, and shared income. It was only under those precise circumstances that he'd consider having a child.

Traffic came to a dead halt. With one hand on the steering wheel, I turned to face Elwin. He was gazing out the front window, his hands in his lap, his caramel skin lightly dotted with freckles, his breathing shallow. Elwin was the first Black man I'd loved this passionately, the only one who made me rethink my priorities, choose a different adventure. He introduced me to polyamory, gave me the language of my salvation from toxic monogamous relationships I could never quite make work. He taught me about politics, Black flight, and reproductive justice. When I first met him—drunk at a conference dance party in 2015—I knew without knowing his name that if I didn't keep his attention, I'd regret it for the rest of my life.

Elwin noticed me staring at him and made eye contact. "What?"

"I thought you *wanted* to get married and have children."

He scoffed. "No way! I can't be someone's daddy."

That was the moment. This man I loved enough to change my relationship style for was the first—read: only—man with whom I wanted to have children. His love was all-consuming, and I drowned in him willingly. Whenever I imagined my future, my children were his. My height, his freckles, our smarts. I honestly couldn't fathom a world in which I would give birth to any other man's children. I still can't.

But when he told me didn't want to have kids, that he didn't want to be the biological parent to anyone's child, which included mine, the daughter, with fresh twists and a smile so wide she could charm fascists, died inside me. I felt her vanish, not ripped away from my arms so much as her image turned cloudy, then faded entirely. I see bits of her in my friends' children now, but I could never put her back together. Her name was Angela.

Traffic started moving again. I lingered on Elwin for a moment more, then eased off the brake to take us home.

When we broke up, it was tumultuous. The most explosive breakup of my lifetime. I grieved for our relationship, but mostly I grieved the future he'd promised we would never have. I'd have to rebuild it in my own image.

***

My first gynecologist approved the surgery. He told me the recovery was about two weeks, and I needed to make sure I could do that. The only way I could swing that was if I had the procedure done during winter or summer break. As a stopgap, he offered me birth control pills. I didn't like the side effects, and I'd just started seeing Rob, so we were doing little else than having sex, and I didn't want to chance forgetting a pill, therefore rendering this entire exercise moot.

He offered the IUD. I agreed.

Two months or so later, I sat in an examination room, waiting for my birth control implant to be removed. My original gynecologist had transferred to exclusively labor and delivery, so I was assigned someone new. The nurse came in and told me they couldn't do both procedures—removing my implant and inserting my IUD—during the same visit. Something about my insurance. Which did I want done today?

I rolled my eyes. "The implant, I guess." The doctor came in then, Dr. M., we'll call her, and asked me why I was getting these procedures done.

"I don't want to have kids," I told her. "Just not in the cards for me."

"But what if you meet a man who wants to marry and have kids with you?" she asked.

My imagined daughter flashed across my eyes. "I've already met him, and he doesn't want kids either." *What an inappropriate question*, I thought. "Besides, this is just a stopgap until I can schedule my sterilization surgery."

Dr. M. blinked at me. "My daughter says she doesn't want kids, either, but getting your tubes tied feels a bit much." She took back my paperwork and sighed. "Oh, well." She left the room to get the nurse who would help her extract my implant.

I didn't want to discuss my recurring nightmares surrounding pregnancy, how likely I am to die from childbirth complications because medical professionals assume all women in general, and Black women specifically, to be hysterical (see: etymology of "hysterectomy") and therefore unreliable reporters of their own symptoms, of their own bodies (see: the medical team that almost killed Serena Williams on the birthing table because they didn't believe her when she said something was wrong).

Any woman afraid of pregnancy is immature, and if I don't want children, I'm selfish.

***

Twenty-four hours after I had my implant removed, Election Day 2020—where were *you*?—I sat in the same examination room, awaiting my IUD insertion, reading a book of poetry.

In this moment, I became aware, suddenly and with shocking precision, that though I trust women because I want women to trust me, White women often forget to return the favor.

My doctor—well, the physician performing my procedure—was White. On principle, she gave me information, but perhaps, also on principle, she withheld it. I've read that cervical grazes can be pleasurable during penetrative sex, but usually only during total arousal (see: tenting). Under every other circumstance, touching the cervix for a biopsy (see: colposcopy), childbirth (see: natural or vaginal birth), or routine procedures (see: IUD insertion or removal, Pap smear, diaphragm or birth control ring insertion or replacement) will cause nerve endings on the cervix to jolt and spasm—resulting in pain.

The IUD is placed inside the uterus, a plastic or copper T with strings that hang out of the cervix. To insert it, one might dilate the cervix through medication, then navigate the device into the uterus. The nurse kept telling me to relax, stop tensing, as my vision blurred and reset, my pulse rapid and inconsistent, my breathing erratic. I'd had cramps that brought me to my knees before, but this was like my uterus found throwing stars and C-4 to tear down her own walls.

Tsking to herself afterward, Dr. M. said she should have told me to take pain medication before coming in today. I couldn't muster the energy to fix my face from the pure incredulous hatred aimed squarely at her. She was lucky we were both masked.

The trouble with White women is that often they think it unnecessary to listen to or believe women of color, Black women especially. Like how the #MeToo movement was started ten years before by a Black woman, but only gained credence and momentum when White women started using the hashtag. Or how Susan B. Anthony would rather give up her right arm before she'd support the vote for the Negro before the woman. I kept hearing Dr. M.'s question—*What if you meet a man who wants to marry and have kids with you?*—and the harm tensed every nerve in my body. I'm supposed to play fast and loose with my pussy in case an imaginary man wants my genes in his offspring? No. I became dizzy, clenching muscles I couldn't name, trying to protect myself from that inappropriate commentary. I struggled to breathe deeply, sweat beading my forehead, my nails carving half moons into my palms.

The body's failsafe for protection is its memory—it remembers everything, but if I try now to recall the sensation of my uterus contracting around a foreign object, I fail. I couldn't relax an internal organ, couldn't breathe through her panic attack, quell her fight-or-flight response with stillness and calm. My womb had been under siege for over a decade—rape after rape, birth control after Plan B, irregular period after STD, plus an actual miscarriage—and she was tired of this permanent self-defense posture.

Me too, honey, me too.

The medical team left me in the examination room alone, the lights off but for a small lamp on the desk. I pressed my belly and imagined my uterus planning an escape. Conspiring with the ovaries and fallopian tubes, she marched back and forth in the war room of my lower abdomen, demanding swift and severe action, the IUD the last straw to break her. How dare I plant a cross inside her, tell her she can't make a baby, can't renovate, can't clean up nice? If I'm not careful, she won't burn it; she'll bury it and take me with her.

I wish my White woman physician had told me to take ibuprofen for my uterus's temper tantrum, to apply a heating pad for when she calmed down, to take the rest of the day off so we could both recover and apologize to each other. When I asked at the start of this if there was anything I should know, she told me no. I believe in the end she considered me dramatic, exaggerating the pain scale since it's normal to experience cramps after this procedure.

Silly girl, you must be overreacting.

Did my doctor's level of care change when she discovered I wanted sterilization? When a doctor labels a patient *selfish*, does she become a sadist? Was it easier to dilate the cervix of a thirty-year-old Black woman who's never had children *without* medication because I deserve *some* pain if I'm going to skip the miracle of childbirth?

During sex, my partner slaps my ass and fucks me hard, supplying pain I crave, am desperate for. This pleasure is about power—how I can request to be hurt but not harmed, stung not stabbed, smarting not suffering. Even in my consent to receive treatment, evidenced by my signature, I did not give permission to be dismissed, only offered information when pleaded for, or tortured at the hands of a White woman on Election Day.

I am not a purchased experiment to forward modern medicine. She is not J. Marion Sims reincarnated.

I expect betrayal from faceless White women drunk on their own subjugation, aching for relevance in the patriarchy that alleges to protect them as it deprives them of pleasure and relevance—but I want to trust my attending physician, even if she is White, even if she doesn't agree with my decision to remain childless, even if she has given me no reason to trust her.

I want to leave better than when I arrived.

Shivering on that examination table, lights out, my knees locked together, I couldn't slow my heart rate enough to get up, get dressed, and walk out of there. My womb cramped in time to a question I've never asked out loud—*when will I feel safe again?*—and I forced myself to stand.

Vision still a bit blurry, I slid off the examination table and grabbed my jeans. Breathing like a woman in a Lamaze class, I got dressed, put on my shoes, and stumbled out of the building. No one paid any attention to me, my checkout already completed, and I shuddered across the parking lot to a bench, where I collapsed.

With one hand on my belly, I ripped off my mask and called my soon-to-be husband, Rob, who had walked me to the clinic in the first place. It hurt to speak. I managed a few words—*pain, too much, come get me*—before simply hanging up and bursting into tears.

I don't remember getting in the car, or entering his apartment, or changing clothes. A few hours later, I woke up drenched in sweat, the cramping finally slowed to a halt.

For days, my womb launched missiles and planted land mines. The cramps would appear and return without warning. How I managed to teach any of my classes is a miracle of triple the recommended dosage of Advil, caffeine pills, and sitting during my lectures instead of standing. When the election results finally came in on that Saturday, the pain had ceased.

**

Weeks later, when I called to cancel my follow-up appointment because I'd contracted COVID-19 and couldn't think straight, the receptionist asked if there was anything else she could do for me.

I looked at the slip of paper in my hand. I had started writing notes to myself to keep from forgetting things—when grades were due, whom to email back, what appointments I needed to make or unmake and what to say when I did so. (COVID kicked my ass, y'all.) "Uh, yeah, can you remove someone from my care team?"

"Oh," she said, surprised. "Well, sure. Who would you like removed?"

"Dr. M."

"Your attending for the IUD procedure?"

"Yes." I crumpled the paper into a small ball and threw it across the room toward nothing. Last thing on the list.

"Right, okay. Yes, she's been removed from your care team." She paused. "Is there anything else I can do for you?"

"No, thank you, have a nice day."

I want to believe the mistake of not advising me to take pain meds and not prescribing me a medication to dilate my cervix were just that—mistakes. I don't want to make this incident about race. But on Election Day, with a Black woman running as VP, with the country's future on the backs of Philadelphia and Black voters? The 53 percent of White women who voted for Trump looms in my memory—which White woman was Dr. M. that day? And why do I live in a world where that distinction could potentially kill me?

No one believes Black women experience pain—just look how strong we are, always have had to be.

***

In 2021, a year after I got my IUD, I scheduled an appointment with my now third gynecologist to get my triannual Pap smear. Dr. S., we'll call her—still White because of course—entered the room with an Asian woman who was shadowing her after the nurse left. We talked briefly about my history and why I was there.

"I need a Pap smear, but I also want to talk about scheduling my sterilization surgery," I said, flexing my toes in my ballet flats. It was late October, the weather unseasonably dry.

"Why do you want to have your tubes removed?"

We went through the whole thing again, but I must have been less convincing this time. "My original physician approved this surgery already," I said. "Is there a reason I have to do this again?"

"Well..."

The biggest concern doctors have when arranging a tubal ligation (the "tying off" of the fallopian tubes) or salpingectomy (the removal of one or both tubes) is what Dr. S. called "the risk of regret." My age—under forty—and medical history—mostly healthy aside from long-COVID symptoms that had rendered me unable to teach that semester—combined with my race—Black AF—and polyamorous lifestyle made me especially "high-risk for regretting [my] choice down the line," Dr. S. explained.

"But you seem resolved, and it's in your file that you've asked for this already," Dr. S. said quickly after I stared at her for several seconds silently. "I just need to consult with the attending surgeon, and then we'll decide."

In the meantime, I prepared for the Pap smear. Not having it every year put me out of practice, so unsure if this included a breast exam, I got completely undressed and sat on the examination table.

When Dr. S. returned, she brought her shadow, the nurse from before, and the attending surgeon—the first Black woman I'd seen in the hospital. Dr. W., the surgeon, asked if I wanted to have this conversation after the Pap smear, since I was naked, but I declined. "Let's just get this over with," I said.

Dr. W. explained that she would not approve the surgery. "I used to feel exactly like you before I had kids," she said.

No, you couldn't have, because I still don't want to have kids.

She noted that my anxiety about being pregnant or giving birth wasn't a good enough reason to approve my request. "What about having children is so stressful to you?" she asked.

I looked her directly in the eyes, pressing that crinkly paper against my chest. "I cannot take any of the vicarious grief I experience when Black children are shot dead in the streets; I will not survive it if one day it's my child."

No one spoke for a moment. I looked at the ceiling, tears welling up in my eyes.

"I think you should wait a little longer," Dr. W. finally said. "The IUD is working great, so no need to also have the surgery."

I shook my head and didn't meet her gaze. Betrayal by the only woman in the room who understood what I meant stung the back of my throat.

"Do you understand?"

"Yeah." I swallowed hard.

Dr. W. left, and they completed my Pap smear quickly. "Go ahead and get dressed, and we'll call you if your results come back abnormal; otherwise, you're free to go," Dr. S. said. I nodded. She lingered in the room for a bit, almost as if she wanted to apologize, but then she left with the others.

I got dressed and went to the checkout station. "Did they want you to schedule a follow-up?" the receptionist asked.

"I doubt it, they didn't do anything," I almost shouted. Not wanting to get involved—smart—the receptionist wished me a good day and I left.

In the car, I started sobbing. I was going to live in this fear, this grief for a child I will never have and the one I didn't realize I'd lost for the rest of my life. Simply because someone who isn't in my body gets to decide whether I deserve to carry this pain.

At home, Rob cooked dinner while singing along to his own music. When he saw me, he shut it off, and I cried in his arms, the pasta water boiling over.

***

A week after Drs. S. and W. denied my surgery, Dr. S. called me. My Pap smear results were normal, and she told me that she'd thought over what I said during our appointment. "I think you are right," she said, "so I'm approving the surgery. I'll have our OR nurse call you to schedule it."

"Thank you."

"Of course."

Finally, after three doctors and one canceled appointment due to staff shortages, I sat in a hospital bed, stomach empty. My surgeon, Dr. O., was an Indian man with kind eyes. He and the rest of the surgical team explained the risks and recovery time, and had me sign a bunch of paperwork. I kept making everyone laugh, which made it hard to find a vein for my fluids. Rob sat next to me playing his Switch. We had recently gotten engaged. He was responsible for me if anything went wrong, and his anxiety was through the roof, but he played it cool.

Hours later, I woke up in recovery with no pain, surprisingly. That whole week was easy—I never had any pain, and the surgical scars healed quickly. It would take another year for them to remove my IUD, but for the first time since I was eighteen, I felt safe. Finally.

I don't see my imagined daughter anymore. Maybe she was just me reflected, wanting someone to save her, to protect her. Maybe she was a reminder that I *am* reliable when it comes to my body, my future. Maybe she was a sign to leave that man who would be her father, to dodge the bullet before it left the chamber.

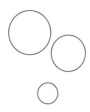

A Weight Too Heavy

Leah Mueller

I scrambled up the slippery bank toward my waiting train. Half-bare patches of January snow dotted the hillside like dirty stubble. A series of ice storms had recently plagued the region. After a brief thaw, subzero temperatures refroze the melted water into a brittle shell. My cheap boot soles clawed at the earth, then slid backward toward the sidewalk.

The train let out an impatient belch of steam. It was scheduled to leave Evanston at 9:34, but I was half a minute late. I heaved myself onto the platform and landed in front of a set of sliding doors. The aperture remained open long enough for me to squeeze inside.

Panting hard, I staggered toward an empty seat. Most of Evanston's workforce had already started their shifts. My body felt much heavier than usual. Something hard was lodged in the pit of my belly. Perhaps the remnants of my previous night's dinner. I couldn't even remember what I'd eaten.

The train blew its whistle and shuddered, then lurched forward. It gradually picked up momentum, passing immaculate homes and tidy lines of parked cars. I gazed out the window at the pastoral scene. Filthy rich, all of them. Not a worry in the world.

How did people manage to get their hands on that much money? Most of them were born into wealth. Lucky bastards.

I closed my eyes and tried to ignore the disturbance in my belly. The ponderous object kept shifting, like a board angling for a flush surface. I placed a hand beneath my coat and caressed my stomach with the tip of one finger. The skin felt as swollen as an overripe melon, though I hadn't gained a pound since high school.

I didn't have time to worry. I'd agreed to paint an acquaintance's Winnetka apartment. She'd promised to provide brushes, rollers, and a drop cloth, plus $200 after completion. Kelly was a pleasant but clueless woman who didn't know how to paint walls. Her parents had purchased the place only a few weeks beforehand.

The end door whooshed open, and a uniformed conductor strolled into the aisle. He cleared his throat, tapped my armrest, and smiled. "Your fare please." I reached into my purse and pulled out a ticket. The conductor gave it a perfunctory glance, then punched a small hole in the center. After attaching the stub to the back of my seat, he strolled away in search of other passengers.

I'd always found this ritual comforting. It reminded me of taking the train to Wisconsin to visit my grandmother. After I turned eleven, my parents let me go by myself. "She's so independent," everyone said. I scrutinized each station with care, making sure I knew exactly how many stops remained until my destination.

Leaning against the window, I tried my hardest to get comfortable. I could feel the cold glass through my winter coat. The chill soothed my queasiness, but only for a moment. Outside, the houses kept getting fancier. Enormous porches, some with columns. Park-like front yards, half covered in snow. Quaint shops selling leisure outfits to people who didn't know how to relax.

The train left the outskirts of Evanston and headed north through Wilmette. Finally, it screeched to a halt in Winnetka. I rose unsteadily from my seat and wandered toward the platform. My head spun from a debilitating combination of nausea and vertigo.

Perhaps eating would help. As usual, I'd skipped breakfast. My boyfriend was a restless sleeper, so I'd awakened several times in the middle of the night. Scott worked sporadically at odd jobs, only showing up if somebody phoned him. The rest of the time, he stayed in bed as much as possible.

I found a deli named Beautiful Food and wandered inside. Gleaming glass bowls overflowed with a variety of elaborate salads. Figs, grapes, arugula, pine nuts. Everything looked gorgeous, like a magazine cover. Above the display, a sign read, "Daily special! Three Salad Sampler, $20.00."

Twenty bucks was a ridiculous sum for three scoops of salad. I wasn't certain if I could eat that much. Still, I needed to shove some calories into my heaving belly if I expected to spend eight hours inhaling paint fumes.

My eyes had a hard time focusing on the cuisine options. A middle-aged female cashier stared at me without expression. Her hair and makeup looked impeccable. Perhaps she was a wealthy North Shore matron who only worked at Beautiful Food as a hobby. The afternoons were long in Winnetka.

"Can I answer any questions about our salads?" she asked.

What kind of question could I possibly have about salads? I shook my head and pointed toward one of the bowls. Its contents featured artichoke hearts and shaved carrots. "I'll take that one. And the couscous mix. And the one with broccolini."

A fresh spasm of nausea overwhelmed me as I trudged toward my table. I set down my tray and clasped the back of my chair with both hands. Cramps rocketed through my gut, almost knocking me to the floor. It felt like someone had taken a chainsaw to my stomach. What the hell was going on? Maybe I had food poisoning. I'd never felt so sick in my life.

The cashier remained in her spot behind the counter. Eyes downcast, she rubbed a clean rag around the edge of a salad bowl. Her face looked expressionless, as if nothing out of the ordinary was happening.

"Do you have a restroom I could use?" I could barely choke out the words.

For the first time, the woman smiled. Her milk-white teeth were straight and perfect, like a freshly painted picket fence. "Certainly," she replied, to my immense relief. "It's in the back." She gestured toward the opposite wall.

The tiny bathroom reeked of lavender air freshener. I staggered toward the toilet, unzipped my jeans, and pulled down my underwear. Perching on the edge of the seat, I cradled my head in my palms. Cold sweat trickled between my fingers. I rocked back and forth, trying to soothe the undulating cramps.

An enormous, dark-red clot emerged from my vagina and plopped into the bowl. Half the size of one of my fists, it sank to the bottom of the toilet and broke apart. A cascade of smaller clots followed. Then a second one, and a third. The meaty clumps swirled together in the crimson water.

I stared at the carnage and tried not to panic. The good citizens of Winnetka would probably put me in a straitjacket. Or they'd call an ambulance, and I'd be stuck with a medical bill I couldn't afford to pay. Either way, I was fucked.

Eight weeks had passed since my last period. Perhaps nine. Normally, I could set a clock by my menstrual cycle, but I'd stopped paying attention. My IUD caused so many infections that I'd asked a doctor to yank it five years beforehand. I figured the device had rendered me infertile. Despite all the sex I'd experienced, no seed ever implanted itself inside my body.

Besides, I was too stressed out to care. Scott and I fought constantly, and our erotic life suffered as a result. Stress could stop periods in their tracks, but this wasn't a normal period. Usually, the blood started as an almost imperceptible trickle and gradually increased in volume. The toilet contained more blood than I shed in a week.

My mind did back flips as I struggled to accept the truth. I was having a miscarriage. The bowl held a microscopic fetus and some torn lining from my uterus. For whatever reason, my body didn't see fit to complete its nine-month gestation. The tiny speck would never become a human being.

I felt no grief whatsoever. Only emptiness, a void so deep that I could do nothing but stare at the bowl. None of it seemed real. I hovered above a restaurant toilet in one of the richest towns in America, watching the remnants of my pregnancy dissolve into the water.

Bracing a hand against the sink, I staggered to my feet. My head spun, but only for a moment. I mopped at my vagina with a wad of toilet paper until all the bloody residue was gone. Then I flushed everything away, like none of it had ever existed.

After emerging from the bathroom, I glanced around the deli. The cashier remained at her post behind the register. My untouched plate rested on the table, as if awaiting my return. I shuffled toward a chair. At least the terrible cramping had vanished. My body seemed impossibly light, like it was in danger of toppling at any moment.

The salad piles looked enormous, intimidating. No way in hell could I eat all that food. Still, I'd paid twenty bucks for my goddamn meal. I needed to choke down a few mouthfuls, even if they tasted like wads of soggy newspaper.

Swallowing felt like torture. I drifted into a silent pit of self-recrimination. Somehow, my uterus knew I was unfit to be a mother. Scott and I would make awful parents. The burden of childrearing was too heavy for us. We could barely look after ourselves. Despite my body's obvious clues, I hadn't even realized I was pregnant. Weren't women supposed to intuit such things?

I glanced at the wall clock. 11:30. Barely enough time for me to dump the remainder of my food and arrive at Kelly's place by noon. She finished work at 6:00, so I would need to split my painting into two shifts. That meant a second trip to Winnetka and an extra train ticket. Rent day loomed ahead, less than a week away.

Though I felt exhausted, I couldn't afford to go home early. Naps were a luxury for people who could afford them. I shoveled my leftovers into a trash can, zipped my coat, and headed for the door. A nearby wall thermometer read ten degrees. I hoped I could walk fast enough to stay warm. If I kept moving forward, everything would be okay.

The street seemed even noisier than usual. Three more blocks, and I'd be in the sanctuary of Kelly's apartment. I'd dip a clean roller into a paint tray and forget that I'd just had a miscarriage. Indulging my distress was an exercise in futility. I still had so much work to do, and never enough rest to make up for it.

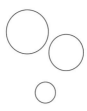

On Being So-Called Sensitive

Chloe Caldwell

When my friend Morgan and I first heard about the fertility drug Clomid, we looked at each other wide-eyed. I was in my desperate era. We were at Rivertown Lodge in Hudson, a bougie hotel where she was staying while visiting me, and sitting across from one another with open laptops. We were trying to compare the lab results of our AMH (the amount of eggs you have) and FSH (follicle-stimulating hormone) and decode shit. We had no clue how to read these charts; we were both at the beginning of what would turn into longish fertility journeys. We had no idea what we were doing. But Clomid! Was it a miracle drug? Another friend, Taryn, had told me about it; she'd been on the edge of taking it when she had not conceived in two years. She was worried, though, about the risk of multiples. Luckily, she got pregnant naturally before she had to take it. I told Morgan this, how the "superovulation" blows up the ovaries, and instead of the one mature follicle we usually drop a month, Clomid can make two, three, even six mature follicles.

"It's like a shortcut," Taryn explained, "Then you get two kids in one shot!" It was all abstract to us; when you want a baby and haven't conceived in a year or two, the idea of actually getting two babies seems impossible. A joke, even.

My gynecologist has done all my fertility tests and deemed everything normal. When I brought up Clomid hopefully, he explained he wouldn't prescribe it to me since I already ovulated normally, and Clomid was more helpful for people with PCOS, as it would induce ovulation in anovulatory people.

Okay. Fair.

But the fertility clinic was another story. Their treatment plan for me was four rounds of Clomid along with an IUI (intrauterine insemination).

By now, I'd read a little about what the internet called the "Clomid crazies"(which is a stupid cutesy term meant to downplay the severity of dysphoria, rage, and suicidal thoughts). I could handle it, I decided. I'd conquered having premenstrual dysphoric disorder (PMDD)! Yes, I'd had a bad reaction when I took birth control ten years ago and was thinking about guns and bullets. But this was different; I wanted a baby, right? So woman the heck up and do it.

Clomid is to be taken for five consecutive days, usually starting on day three of your menstrual cycle and ending on day seven. I took it before bed—everyone said that way you'd sleep through the side effects. I was okay the first couple of days, but on the final day, a horrible, terrifying rage and dissociation came over me. One moment I held my favorite blue ceramic mug full of peppermint tea; the next thing I knew, I'd smashed it into pieces in one (impressive) throw against the wall. Again, this was my favorite mug.

Before that, I'd been lying on the couch, and a gross feeling came over me. There was a voice in my head telling me never to take Clomid again. It's hard to describe the way Clomid made me physically and emotionally feel, but the word that comes up is "creepy." Creepy as fuck. When my then-partner, Tony, came upstairs, I told him I would never take this drug again (isn't it funny how doctors call it "medicine"?).

I was praised by the nurses for how "well" I'd done on Clomid. I'd produced four mature follicles! They were big! Like 22mm big! "You took really well to the medicine," the nurse told me, pleased.

Cut to me absolutely going against my instincts and taking it again. There's the voice though, the pathetic, desperate voice who wants the baby. Those twins I was promised. Should I pull up my bootstraps, ruin my marriage, and become a shell of who I used to be to get them? Sure, I'd thrown my favorite mug against the wall near my husband, screaming, but otherwise I'd been fine! Don't be a pussy. Be a good girl and take the medicine. Woman up.

Round two of Clomid: Have you ever looked in the mirror during an acid or psilocybin trip and suddenly your face looked like a Picasso painting? Clomid made me psychotic, and I am not speaking in hyperbole. I began screaming I had no control of my life; my voice changed, my hand didn't look like it was really my hand. I walked from room to room, moaning, sobbing, hyperventilating. Panicking. I felt creepy again, and this time, I could actually feel my ovaries tingeing and growing, and it felt so unnatural. If they say giving birth is the most natural thing in the world, well, Clomid is the opposite.

In my notes app:

Clomid diaries
Day 3
A blood moon last night
Storm today
Full moon tonight
I'm in the thick of it
Help

Tony encouraged me to record a voice memo. We were sitting in our bed, with the lights off. It reminded me of the *before* days; before I knew what Clomid was, when we'd take the occasional MDMA, and we'd be in the bedroom in the middle of the day. God, I missed that.

After describing my Clomid trip to Tony, and having a long talk, I decided to throw the rest of the pills away, exactly how I had with birth control ten years ago. Tony had said something about how Clomid was the opposite of what we think of when we think of making a baby: love, trust, orgasm. Instead we were in pain, distrust, violence.

I don't go into medical treatments blindly. I read a ton, outsource, possibly to the point of detriment. I thought I'd read enough about Clomid. I was wrong. It wasn't until I came out of my Clomid psychosis, and after a friend asked me if I thought Clomid was worse for me since I struggled with PMDD, that I googled it:

> The side effect profile reported by some women using clomiphene citrate is similar to symptoms of premenstrual dysphoric disorder (PMDD), including tension, irritability, depressed mood, affective lability, lack of energy, difficulty concentrating, and physical symptoms such as breast tenderness, bloating, headache.

Wait. So Clomid induced PMDD psychosis in patients? Shouldn't someone have asked me in advance what my history of PMDD and PMS was? Shouldn't I have been warned, informed, so I could make a responsible decision? Shouldn't they have seen from my medical records that I had a PMDD diagnosis? This all could have been avoided, especially since there is another drug called letrozole, which essentially does the same thing as Clomid, but apparently, since I was over thirty-five, they defaulted to Clomid.

When I wrote to the clinic and told them my reaction to Clomid, they wanted to set up a phone meeting. I appreciated the gesture and had it on speaker phone so Tony could listen in. The doctor agreed I should not use Clomid again, though of course it was a shame since, again, I "took so well to the medicine." I hadn't even taken all five pills, but I still had four mature follicles again, even bigger this time. She admitted she was stumped on why I wasn't getting pregnant.

The conversation was mostly helpful, until the end when the doctor said I must be "really sensitive to Clomid. Most people are fine," she said.

I'd beg to differ. I'd just gotten off a bender of watching Clomid TikToks and reading both Reddit and academic articles and studies:

Clomid Is the Devil Drug (posted on The Bump)
Clomid Is the Devil in Disguise (posted on Glow)
Clomid Is the Devil (posted on TikTok)
Clomid Side Effect: Suicidal Thoughts (posted on eHealthMe)
Clomifene: Suicidal Ideation[1]
Clomiphene Citrate as a Possible Cause of a Psychotic Reaction
    During Infertility Treatment[2]
Psychotic Reaction Associated with Clomiphene-Induced Ovulation[3]
Mental Health Issues on Clomid (posted on Reddit)
Clomid-Induced Psychosis[4]

> From Reddit:
>
> My husband likes to rate my Clomid cycles like they rate spicy dishes at a Chinese restaurant ("Can I get it two-pepper hot?") He tells my doctor, "This cycle was 'two-divorce' bad; she wanted to get a divorce only twice this time."

So yeah, maybe I'm *sensitive*. Or maybe *not*, since hundreds of *thousands* of other women have apparently experienced this as well. Maybe it's time to research women's health. Maybe it's time to ask patients about their history with mental health, PMS, and PMDD before giving out a drug that induces psychosis and suicidal ideation to people who are already struggling with the hell of infertility, which is a life crisis in itself.

It's not up to me if you take Clomid. Hopefully you'll be one of the lucky ones. Just clear your house of anything ceramic and maybe lock yourself in a dark room for five days. And I do not mean that in a cutesy way.

Here's the kicker: Over a year later, I went to a naturopath doctor. She told me that maitake mushroom tincture does the exact same thing Clomid does, but without side effects. Unfortunately, I learned that when it was too little too late.

I'm grateful to Clomid, though, as it got me listening to my body. The synthetic horse shit hormones or whatever the hell is in there—I'm not a doctor—showed me exactly how my body is not supposed to feel. If that's what being sensitive is, then I'll take it.

Notes

1. Anonymous, "Clomifene: Suicidal Ideation," *Reactions Weekly*: Auckland 1571 (October 3, 2015), 60.
2. F. Siedentopf, B. Horstkamp, G. Stief, and H. Kentenich, "Clomiphene Citrate as a Possible Cause of a Psychotic Reaction During Infertility Treatment," *Human Reproduction* 12, no. 4 (April 1, 1997): 706–7, https://doi.org/10.1093/humrep/12.4.706.
3. K. Hazuki, I. Satoshi, T. Hiroshi, K. Ichiro, I. Atsushi, et al., "Psychotic Reaction Associated with Clomiphene-Induced Ovulation," *Bio-Medical Journal of Scientific & Technical Research* 17, no. 3 (April 2019), 12793–4, https://doi.org/10.26717/BJSTR.2019.17.002996.
4. "Clomid-Induced Psychosis," Letters to the Editor, *Psychiatry Online*, American Psychiatric Association, https://psychiatryonline.org/doi/pdf/10.1176/ajp.154.8.1169b.

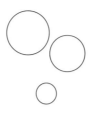

Monsters
An Excerpt from *Knocked Down: A High-Risk Memoir*

Aileen Weintraub

After coming home from one final pre-baby-making trip to Costa Rica just a few short months into married life, I cornered my husband Chris in front of the pantry where he was crunching through a box of crackers.

"We're going to make a baby!"

"Right now? I have to go to work."

I swatted him on the shoulder. "Not now. I'm just telling you so you can prepare whatever it is you have to prepare."

"Right. What am I preparing? Do you want me to lift weights? This sounds hard." His head still in the pantry, I could see crumbs forming in a pyramid on the floor.

"Just make sure your boys have a lot of breathing room, okay? Is there enough ventilation under your desk at work?"

"Don't worry, they're safe." He kissed me and headed out the door.

"I'm serious," I yelled after him, but he was gone.

On New Year's Eve Chris came home with the flu. I made sure he stayed hydrated and was getting enough to eat because

I cared deeply for his well-being, but I'm not going to lie—I was ovulating. I plied him with champagne and made a small attempt at sexy talk, but I could tell I was losing him, and even when our lovemaking reached a fever pitch, I knew his flushed face was because his temperature was rising and not because of my sexual prowess. Luckily, inebriated and sick as he was, Chris was a willing accomplice.

Two weeks later I was standing tall and strong in Warrior One pose during a Sunday morning yoga class, arms reaching to the sky, my lower half grounded toward the earth. Suddenly my legs began to twitch; my flesh tingled. My stomach growled, loudly. People were looking at me. A wave of warmth rushed over me, rising up and enveloping me as though a supernatural force was taking hold. I didn't have to pee on a stick. I didn't scramble to make a doctor's appointment. I knew. After a few more weeks passed, I called my ob-gyn.

At the appointment, the nurse marveled at how calm and self-assured I was. I had no questions and I wasn't nervous, which was unusual given my penchant for worrying as a pastime. I was on a good and steady course, not giving in to my cravings, cutting back on the caffeine, giving up wine and martinis, and maintaining a healthy diet. I even earmarked pages in what I called the "baby bibles" for Chris to read. Every appointment since my first had gone off without a hitch.

At eighteen weeks I came home from a long day of walking around Manhattan with Chris. I was feeling an unusual pain in my lower belly, so I called the nurse. She told me not to worry and that I should wait for my already scheduled appointment the next day to address my concerns with the doctor.

The exam began in the usual way with the nurse asking questions and taking my blood pressure. When the doctor walked in and said hello, the first thing I noticed was the curve of her lips. They glistened with a red sheen that was painted on so precisely I knew she must touch up her lipstick between patients. I told her about my pain and she asked to examine me, Chris sitting by my side.

A few moments later, caught up in my own reverie, I could not make sense of what the doctor was trying to tell me; I could only register the fact that my baby might fall out of my uterus at any moment. My vision began to blur and both Chris and the doctor seemed far away, her voice echoing like she was down a rabbit hole. I was rushed into an emergency sonogram. Chris squeezed into the corner of the small room. I arched my neck back, compelled to see the screen behind me, as if I could diagnose the problem on my own.

"Wow, um. Okay," said the sonographer, Sherry. She moved her magic wand around my belly and looked at the ultrasound screen. "Let's just measure these." A veil of professionalism swept over her face. I'd seen that look on television shows before, when the nurse lifts the sheets and sees mangled and irreparable body parts.

"What do you see?" I asked, not sure I wanted to know.

"You've got some pretty big fibroids in there. No one ever mentioned this to you?"

"It hasn't come up in conversation." I waited, expecting more, but she said nothing. As she was printing out the scans, the doctor reappeared and said that I had two football-sized fibroids and another tennis ball–sized one growing in my uterus, and because they were so big, they were pressing up against some vital things in there. I don't know if she was exaggerating their size or not, but she had made her point. Oh, and one of those vital things was the baby.

Fibroids are noncancerous tumors that look like big, meaty, bulbous growths. They are a bit reminiscent of that old movie The Blob where the amoeba-like alien terrorizes a small town, getting bigger and bigger with every victim it consumes. So my uterus had pretty much become the setting of a horror movie.

I'd had no idea I had fibroids before this moment. I feel it's necessary to clarify this point here because every single person I have met since that doctor's appointment, including the doctor, has asked me how it is possible that I didn't know I had fibroids before getting pregnant. But since I had never actually looked inside my own uterus, and no one had ever told me during previous sonograms, I was just as surprised as everyone else to find out.

My fibroids were so astronomically large that Sherry dubbed them the "Monster Fibroids." In all her years she had never seen such large masses competing with a fetus. The doctor explained that one of the Monsters was pressing against my cervix, and the pressure was shortening it to an alarming degree.

The term incompetent cervix was bandied about; as if I didn't have enough self-esteem issues, now my cervix was incompetent. That was like five more years of therapy right there. I'd like to lobby for a name change on this one. How about Independent Cervix That Makes Its Own Decisions About Whom And What It Will Support? All we need to do is throw in hostile uterus, another offensive medical term, and between the two, we'd have the workings of a perfectly dysfunctional marriage. Whatever we chose to call it at the time, the doctor's diagnosis said it all: "There's a good chance you won't be able to support a full-term pregnancy. You'll be tremendously lucky if your baby makes it to twenty-four weeks."

I turned to Chris, who had been sitting quietly as if trying to teleport himself out of the room, and our eyes connected. The color had drained from his face. His full lips formed a flat line but then pursed up on one side. It was too much to bear witness to, and so I averted my gaze. I almost wished he'd scream, get up, ask all the questions, so I wouldn't have to.

I turned back to the doctor, focusing again on her mouth. I no longer saw the rest of her face, just those stop-sign-red lips delivering bad news. Dr. Lipstick was so nonchalant, talking as though she were providing the day's weather forecast, that when I glanced at Chris again he had an expression of utter hatred for this woman. He brought his hands, palms together, up to his mouth and began tapping his fingers.

I was eighteen weeks along, hardly showing my baby bump. The heaviness in my belly was intense, but I couldn't distinguish the physical pain from the emotional. Her words became a jumble as I flashed back to the wintry morning when I had told Chris I was pregnant.

The cars were swooshing by on our unplowed road. Standing before him in the kitchen as he was about to pour his cereal, I whispered in his ear, "We planted a seedling." Chris stopped mid-pour, put down the cereal box, and pulled me toward him. We held on to each other's arms and jumped up and down like two kids out for summer recess.

"Already?

"That fast?"

"One and done, baby."

Grinning, he hugged me. "I didn't think it would be that fast." My normally quiet, reserved husband twirled me around the room and dipped me. We both laughed, shocked and giddy.

But in the doctor's office, with this news, and the way it was presented to us, that memory in the kitchen didn't seem to belong to us anymore. Those were different people full of hope and happiness, and I hardly recognized them. So I put that memory in my pocket for now.

"I don't like her," Chris said dryly when the doctor left us alone, wrapping his arm around me as I got up from the table. I just stared back at him. It was one of the very few times in my life I had ever been speechless.

"I thought I was doing everything right," I mumbled.

"You didn't do anything wrong," Chris replied.

Dinner plans forgotten, we drove home, my husband's strong hand holding my thigh.

Chris and I woke up early the next morning, limbs entangled. "It'll be okay," he reassured me as he prepared breakfast, urging me to eat.

We drove over an hour to Poughkeepsie, New York, to see a specialist. Doctors have a strong need to cover their asses, so the first doctor requested a second opinion. Dr. Lipstick insisted this specialist was the best in the area, and all high-risk pregnancies were referred to him. *High-risk*. It was a term that lingered in the air, like the remnants of an exploded star that can never be pieced back together.

When we were first told a specialist with advanced-tech ultrasound equipment was the next step, I saw money swirling down the toilet. I knew it wasn't what I was supposed to think about, but we had crappy insurance with a high deductible, and specialists tend to charge 250 bucks just to shake hands. It seemed unfair, since I was the one who had to take off all my clothes below the waist; maybe for 250 smackers, the specialist should have to take his clothes off instead. And then, if I liked what I saw, we could go from there.

Dr. Specialist's technician took a fancy picture of my uterus. I could tell that the tech was trying hard to keep her professional demeanor while looking at her screen, but she, like Sherry the sonographer the day before, was horrified. The Monster Fibroids, it turns out, were bigger than the baby.

Dr. Specialist floated in. A gust of wind drifted across the room and the temperature dipped slightly. It was a $250 entrance if I ever saw one. I was almost disappointed to see that his feet did indeed touch the ground. He took off his black-framed glasses and tapped one of the chrome arms against his teeth as he looked over the sonogram pictures. Then he explained to us that eventually there would be a battle of wills when the Monsters would try to suck the blood supply away from the baby, and because the baby was, well, a baby and not a mutant growth, he or she would likely win. (He forgot to mention the excruciating pain this would cause the host uterus.)

The end of this appointment held out more hope than the one the day before, but it wasn't even close to the miracle we had been looking for. We were told that although the largest Monster was pressing against my cervix, and also the baby's head, my cervix was not in as much danger of effacing as Dr. Lipstick had thought. Still, it was a precarious situation, and the message was clear: lie down for the next five months and don't get up. Ever. Well, at least not until the baby starts to crown.

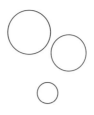

Such a Big Word

Arielle Dance

When I got my first period, I was the perfect mix of overly prepared, embarrassed, and excited. Up to that day, my mother made sure I read books about what to expect of my period, watched videos about being prepared at school, and felt confident peel-and-sticking Always pads with wings to my underwear. What I wasn't prepared for was the physical toll periods would take on my body. I spent the majority of my first period bed-bound—plagued with a low-grade fever, intense cramps, and nightmares. Nearly twenty-five years later, I can still visualize the nightmares—an unfamiliar woman bleeding from her vagina with a snake or big worm in place of her clitoris. I remember waking up from a midday nap drenched in sweat and fearing the bloody worm I'd find on my own body when I went to the bathroom.

I wish I could say that my periods got better from there, but within a year, my periods became more debilitating. I vomited for the first couple of days of every period and even blacked out in some cases. When I'd explain this to friends, they couldn't relate to much beyond the cramping. I couldn't understand how other people were able to go to school during their periods when I had to stay home at least one day per cycle.

After a few years of excruciating periods and heightened symptoms, I started to feel pain between periods. No cause that I could detect, no reason, just sharp pains in my lower abdomen. As a varsity cheerleader and trained dancer, I struggled to balance my extracurriculars with my chronic pain. No longer was the pain isolated to the first few days of my period—instead pain arose at any given time without warning. I would be paralyzed with sharp pains in the midst of a dance class or on the sidelines of a football game. I would be blinded with migraines during an exam. I thought these were growing pains, until I shared the symptoms with my mother. Ever prepared, she opened the most recent edition of *Our Bodies, Ourselves*, scanning for the possible cause of my discomfort. In the early years of WebMD and the peak time to Ask Jeeves, she researched and tried to understand what could possibly be wrong with me.

After countless trips to the emergency room and pediatrician, she took me to a local gynecologist. Each doctor had their own ideas of what could be happening to me—stomach flu, ovarian cysts, and "just bad periods" were all possible culprits. But after birth control failed to improve my symptoms, my mother brought all of her research to my gynecology appointment. She opened *Our Bodies, Ourselves* and said, "I think it's this." She pointed to the page detailing endometriosis. The doctor told my mother it was very unlikely since teenagers, especially Black teenagers, don't really get endometriosis. However, my mother insisted that the doctor perform an exploratory laparoscopy to figure out what may be the issue.

I still remember sitting in a soft white recliner post-op eating crackers and sipping ginger ale when the doctor came in and said, "Well, Mom, you were right." At fifteen years old, my life changed when I was diagnosed with endometriosis. Such a big word for such a young age. Finally, I had answers and a diagnosis. There was something to point to and blame. However, the implications of endometriosis made me fear what a future would be like for me. At fifteen, I heard words like "infertility," "painful sex," and "hysterectomy" before I'd even had my first kiss. While other teenagers were imagining what life would be like when they grew up (college, marriage, family, career, and dreams) I was questioning my future . . . and still in pain.

Over the next ten years, I had numerous surgeries, met with half a dozen gynecologists, and tried every treatment offered in hopes of finding some relief and improved quality of life. Although endometriosis was discovered years before, endometriosis research was still in its infancy during the early 2000s. Gynecologists were prescribing harmful hormone therapies and lacked the skills to surgically excise endometriosis. I was prescribed a monthly injection that suppressed my estrogen and pushed me into a chemical menopause as a teenager. Hot flashes and mood swings were unbearable, and the medication brought no relief to my symptoms.

The month after graduating college, I had my fifth surgery for endometriosis with one of the top specialists in my area. I felt hopeful for some relief and was looking forward to starting a new chapter for my graduate studies. Unfortunately, that summer I developed a pulmonary embolism (blood clot on my lungs). The combination of being sedentary (recovering), having a recent surgery, and being on oral birth control increased my risks for clotting. I have no memory of any doctor warning me about this risk or taking into account that my mother also had a pulmonary embolism while using birth control. What I thought was an asthma attack and gas was actually life-threatening lung trauma. I had shortness of breath and pains in my back that didn't allow me to lie back comfortably.

Again, my mother recognized my symptoms and insisted I go to the emergency room. Based on her experience with blood clots, she feared I may experience the same thing. She was right, again. I spent over a week in the ICU and struggled to regain lung strength.

Being diagnosed with the clot changed my life forever and impacted how I navigated endometriosis treatment. I was no longer able to take estrogen-based medications. An often-ignored aspect of being diagnosed with a blood clot while on birth control is that I had to immediately discontinue taking the Pill while bedbound. When the Pill is discontinued, vaginal bleeding begins quickly. About two days into my stay, my period (or some version of a chemically induced period) began, and I was forced to let nurses change and clean me. For me, this meant being in the ICU, oxygen in my nose, blood thinners and pain medication in my IV, and a bedpan for eliminating... with a period. The cramping and other menstrual symptoms were unbearable, not because of the typical pain, but because of the compounded experiences.

Now, twenty years after my endometriosis diagnosis and fifteen years since that pulmonary embolism, I am still held hostage to my illnesses. That blood clot was not my last; five years later, I was back in the ICU with another pulmonary embolism after a cross-country flight. That fifth surgery was not my last; last year I made the choice to have my uterus removed (keeping my ovaries) to address the debilitating endometriosis and adenomyosis symptoms I was experiencing. I know a hysterectomy is not a cure for endometriosis, but my quality of life has improved significantly. Not having disabling periods is enough of a reason to celebrate. I still feel some twinges of pain every so often, but nothing like before.

Though I'm breathing better and feeling better overall, I recognize how much of my life is still bound to endometriosis and the blood clots. Because I will be on blood thinners for the rest of my life, the way I treat pain will always be impacted—I still cannot take any estrogen-based treatments for any endometriosis that grows back and cannot take certain types of pain medications either. Every doctor's appointment will require a disclosure of my past, and treatments will be planned with that in mind. Nonetheless, I am still grounded in gratitude. I have turned my pain into advocacy and community education about these conditions. And most importantly, it has taught me how to find joy in it all. I love writing about and advocating for people with disabilities; I know that my experiences with pain and illness have shaped the person I am today. And I'm grateful for that.

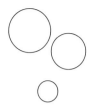

The Five Stages of Out-of-Place Grief

Sammi LaBue

Shock

On Friday before Halloween weekend I was, at long last, pregnant.

I'd taken the day off to prepare for my favorite holiday and to go to my first ultrasound appointment as a pregnant woman. I had seen inside myself dozens of times over the last two-plus years of infertility but had only been met with the gray noise of hormone-grown follicles and the black hole of the large endometrioma in my right ovary. This time I would see the twinkling blip of my growing embryo and "Hear its heartbeat!" as my new pregnancy app had alerted that morning.

But instead, the doctor searched and searched for that fleck of stardust inside me. I could feel the anxiety rise from the frantic movements of her probing wand, could see it on her face growing lines of concern like vines. "We can't find it," she said, the exam room suddenly airless. "We can't hear it."

Denial

I had never heard of an ectopic pregnancy, and the three syllables arrived harshly off the lips of the clinician who confirmed the pregnancy was stuck in my fallopian tube, unviable, and even life-threatening.

The pregnancy inside me was not a baby, could never be. Was only a bit of life blooming in the wrong part of the garden, no sunlight or even moonlight to grow it. Nothing golden with which to attach, to shimmer like the stars we drank to conjure it. My embryo was only six weeks old, but I had already chosen its bedroom paint color, picked the date for a shower, and allocated baby drawers in the kitchen in my mind.

The app I had hastily downloaded, nicknaming my embryo "Moon," was still on my phone, still buzzing at me with prideful announcements in the car home to Brooklyn from the second clinic. "Moon's heart should be starting to beat now!" "Moon's arm buds and eye sockets are developing!" My baby had felt so close after all that time longing to be pregnant—less than eight months away—but instead I ended Friday with three options for its passing: an injection to terminate it, a bloody natural end, or perhaps it would grow too big, rupture my fallopian tube, and send me to the emergency room to avoid death.

The doctor told me to rest. To stay alert to any sudden, acute pain. But I demanded to buy pumpkins, flowers, cobwebs. You can grieve a baby, of course, and even the possibility of one, but what about this? The word "unviable" danced in my head. Could I grieve for what turned out to be a fantasy? The invites for our Halloween party had long been sent out, and so I soldiered on straight into the welcoming fields of distraction.

While I threw myself into pumpkin carving in my kitchen, a text from a friend appeared on my phone. That morning I had sent him an image from the app: "Your baby is the size of a ladybug!" I used my less orange hand to slide his message open. "That's good luck!" he'd replied. I carved into the pulp harder, until my hand blotched red. More dings rang in. *Ladybug emoji.*

Heart. Glitter. Pregnant mother. Baby. At least for someone, it was still as if Moon was only months away from reality.

The next night, I haunted my own Halloween party in the corners of each room, nursing a cocktail I would trade a million times over for the day before to have gone differently.

Anger

That Monday, I was left alone for the first time. After a late and lingering lunch, I detached from my friends like a balloon from a child's wrist, floating directionless, meandering home at dusk.

In my fog I had forgotten that this was actual Halloween. I rounded a corner onto one of the tree-lined brownstone drags of my family-friendly neighborhood and found it teeming with children. A miniature mermaid with an iridescent tail. A round-faced baby lion sporting a toothless smile. A chubby-cheeked Black Panther sucking a pacifier. A veritable parade of babies. It was the family of dinosaurs that undid me. Five dinos in all. Couldn't I have just one?

I ran home to let *Gilmore Girls* babysit me as I have when life is hard since I was a teenager. But suddenly Lorelai complaining about her teenage pregnancy made me want to scream. And I did. Hurling senseless criticism at the television. "It must be so hard having a perfect daughter without even trying!"

Bargaining

The next morning, I fiddled with my baby app again. "Moon has doubled in size in the last week! Grow baby, grow!" I wanted to delete the app, but Moon was still inside me. Sure, the pregnancy was shrinking instead of growing, but ectopic means "out of place," not absent, and I still felt just as pregnant as I had when I first found out.

A few weeks before Halloween, I was at my cousins' house in Bedford, celebrating Canadian Thanksgiving, when I woke up in bed with a smile already on my face. I didn't know what yet, but I felt something shift. It was a good day, and that night my partner and I were the last awake by the outdoor fireplace listening to music. We danced under the moon until we cried for no good reason and every reason at the same time. This is not something we make a habit of, but it was like we were trying to shake free of the loop of fertility disappointment. Tears shined like rivered stars on our cheeks and collected in our open, smiling mouths. We danced for every failure, every missed chance at our dream family, and all the grief that comes with that, not knowing that we had made life until the next day, when the faintest double line appeared in the display of my pregnancy test.

I was so sure this baby that appeared after our moon dance was the one for us that I downloaded the app the day the doctor confirmed the pregnancy. Still, even as my hormone levels dropped, I couldn't delete it knowing Moon was still there.

Depression

After the party and the baby parade, there was nothing left to do but wait. My hormone levels continued going down on their own (the best outcome we could hope for), and suddenly I didn't want to dance or carve pumpkins or yell at Lorelai Gilmore or talk at all. I wanted to sleep and to be still and silent. My husband drove me to Vermont to do that. On our first night in the woods, looking out the bedroom window through my long-faced reflection to the dark trees, I realized I knew this kind of aching want for quiet like I had known the windless shock, the out-of-body anger, the feeling of being pranked that had each made their entrance on cue over the past week. I had been here before. My baby could not ever be a baby, but still, I had met grief again.

Hope

While I waited for my body to heal, people—friends, family, nurses—encouraged me to celebrate. You wanted to be pregnant, and now you have been! But when the blood came, announcing the pregnancy was gone, it felt like death on top of death. Like a dark and moonless night.

On our last day in Vermont after the blood ended, I made an inconsequential joke while doing dinner dishes. "Look at you, being funny," my husband praised before pointing out the fingernail sliver of light in the clear black sky. I had laughed again when the moon was blessedly, inevitably new.

While he donned jacket and gloves for a stargaze, I snuck away to open the app again.

I found the appropriate button: *I have experienced a pregnancy loss.* My thumb wavered in reverence for the dream I thought I might have lived. I closed my eyes and tapped. When I first heard the words "ectopic" and "unviable," I thought they also meant undeserving of grief, but all five stages of loss have surged through me anyway. The app chirped back. "Please take time and care to grieve this loss. We will be here next time."

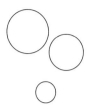

Back at Day One, Again

Abby Koenig

You spend the majority of your adult life desperately trying not to get pregnant. You harness the power of latex and spermicidal creams, sponges and films, pulls and prayers. You spin around in Ortho highs and lows, Yaz, Depo-Provera, vaginal rings. You may be the last living woman on earth to still own a diaphragm.

Up until a certain point in life, babies are just objects to be placed in ladybug costumes in Anne Geddes portraits. For the most part, children don't seem real. They are far away in space and time. Children are unnecessary accessories that celebrities spawn for attention. They scream in the aisles of Target over toys that you've never heard of, with names you can't pronounce. They are cute, yes; you have a nephew that you enjoy sending books to that are well beyond his comprehension. But they are also a time suck and demanding; they smell, and they have green gunk coming out of their noses. Your nephew always finds the perfect time to start crying to his mother, exactly when you are about to tell her something extraordinarily important about your job or your hair. You secretly admit to yourself that you don't even really like children, let alone want one of your own.

The time frame between the place where you have an intense hatred toward the idea of parenting, an "I love my carefree, childless life," an absolute contempt toward people who bring crying babies to brunches and ruin your Bloody Mary buzz to a place where "Oh, that's a cute baby" closes overnight. Literally, it happens as you slumber, going to bed at the young age of twenty-nine and waking up as an old and decrepit thirty-year-old. Now babies don't seem all that bad. You find yourself creepily waving to get their attention in supermarket checkout lines and at shopping malls.

You turn older than thirty, and the seed of fear that has been planted is beginning to blossom. You are a new car that has just driven off the lot; the Blue Book value of your eggs has lessened by 20 percent. Your stock drops a few percentage points every morning that the uterus market opens.

This is the time frame between the "babies are cute" phase and one of utter desperation. You would never expect to turn into one of "those women." You have a career and ambition and a drinking habit, but something in you has changed. You begin to feel a hatred toward all those with children, especially young girls who you just know never wanted their babies to begin with and couldn't possibly love them as much as you could. Jealousy's ugly face looks like yours, and you ain't looking pretty.

Eventually you decide to take action. Your current doctor, whose name is WebMD, has scared you long enough with infertility symptoms and tales of potential cancer stemming from polycystic ovarian syndrome, and so you make an appointment with a real doctor who scares you with tales of polycystic ovarian syndrome (not cancer . . . yet). She can't be sure, though. You are a "nonstandard" case.

You are advised to see a "fertility specialist" who resides in a large, futuristic building labeled with three letters that when placed together in this specific combination have more of a negative connotation than the word "gluten":

IVF

The office takes up an entire floor and has far too many alcoves and evil-looking doors labeled with unwelcoming gold-plated signs reading "In Vitro" and "Family Planning" and "Financial Assistance." Every room has a perfectly positioned box of tissues.

A doctor with impeccably coiffed hair, who is said to be "the best" and whose wall, which is littered with degrees and accolades, backs this up, eyes you up and down. You haven't showered; she must know. She explains your situation, which is to say she has no idea what is wrong with you, but she sounds smart saying it. Regardless of your ailment, she can help. She speaks slowly and deliberately, and after each stanza she asks you if you understand. You nod that yes, yes you do. You leave with a paper in your hand, having absolutely no idea what she just said.

The walls of the IVF clinic are blanketed with photos of smiling babies, which gives you both an idealistic sense of hope and simultaneous dread. They are all twins.

You sit and wait, pants off, to be probed. Despite the apparatus's resemblance to a huge dildo, it is far from an erotic experience. "Cold gel, lots of pressure."

You are given a prescription, pills that will stimulate growth, to be taken on days five through nine, which means nothing considering it has already been established that you have no day one. "We'll just make today day one, then," a bouncy nurse named Jennifer tells you; a scientific approach if you've ever heard one.

The way it is supposed to happen is that you take the pills on the designated days, and then you must return for more probing. If all goes well, meaning your follicles are growing as they should be, on days twelve through fifteen you will have "timed intercourse."

The concept sounds about as romantic as tracking the changing consistencies of your vaginal mucus.

When you go in on day twelve for your probing—"cold gel, lots of pressure"—those damn follicles aren't ready.

"Well, that's surprising!" The nurse tells you, which is surely meant to make you feel good about yourself. You are told that you will have to wait a few more days before you "give yourself the trigger," to which you nod, dumbfounded. Not only do you not know what in the hell the "trigger" is, but you also have an upcoming business trip to Phoenix right when this trigger needs to be . . . well . . . triggered.

The "trigger" is a shot, which you are very nonchalantly told you will need to inject into your own stomach when prompted. The prompt is the exact day you land in Phoenix for a conference on "Fundraising in a Down Economy" being led by you. Lovely.

Your options are limited: bag-check the trigger and pay an obscene fee or find a Walgreens within walking distance of the hotel you are staying at in Phoenix and fill the trigger prescription there. You opt for the cheaper and certainly more risky and awkward option.

Walgreens in Phoenix will have your prescription. They promised, and they texted, but when you get there, they prove to be text-liars. They are dreadfully sorry and will fill the prescription for you tomorrow. Tomorrow, being when you are leading various conference sessions with enthralling titles such as "US Postal Rate Hikes and What That Means to You." Really, who cares?

You suck up all of the pride that you have and tell your male supervisor that you will have to make a swift exit during lunch and will return in "no time." "No time" consists of you hopping a cab, getting to Walgreens, running back to your hotel, shoving a needle into your abdomen, then getting back to the conference to talk about how to milk more money out of unsuspecting schlubs.

You find yourself back at your hotel, needle in hand. You have literally five minutes to self-inject. This is a scary thought. You are a needle virgin. To prepare for the situation, you have bought a box of Band-Aids, rubbing alcohol, gauze, antibacterial cream and a Peppermint Patty (because you fucking deserve it). Oh, and a bag of chips because you deserve those too.

Thank God someone had the foresight to post a video on eHow.com on "how to self-administer an hCG trigger shot." Yes, it is that specific. You slam the needle into your tummy pooch, the only time you've ever been glad to have such a thing, and cold liquid enters your bloodstream, making you slightly nauseous.

Within minutes you are standing before a conference room full of men and women in suits explaining to them, with a monstrously fake smile, how sending reminder letters to donors is a best practice. At the next break, you rush to the bathroom and cry in the stall while shoving the dark chocolate patty down your throat.

While you may think that your untimely egg issue is leveling out, you are sorely mistaken. Recall that you are now "required" to have sex with your husband, who is several thousand miles away, and while he is planning on meeting you in Phoenix, you will be spending the weekend with friends. In their house. Which is one story. And their bedroom is right across the hall.

Quietly timed intercourse, in a friends' guest room, is about as romantic as tracking the changing consistencies of your vaginal mucus and then explaining the process to your husband in full detail.

You silently do the deed, but you know in your heart that nothing good will come of this month's go at it.

And this is your life now. No, not every month is as wildly complicated as the first time, which might have been a good thing in the end. "Well at least we're not in Phoenix," your husband says to you monthly on days twelve through fifteen—sixteen, whatever it happens to be. It's a nice break from the recurring ice of the situation.

Each month that passes becomes more frustrating and lonely. You find it difficult to talk to your friends about the situation, as none of them have children, and most of them aren't even in relationships. You really cannot tell them that you are afraid you are getting too old. The friends who do have children have a confidence that you can't comprehend. "We went through it too," they say, but their success is only a smack in the face at your consistent failure. You try to find solace on infertility message boards, but you find them irritatingly optimistic and filled with annoying acronyms such as TTC, which you had to google.

You make pacts with yourself on every day nine to try harder. You cut out coffee and limit your wine intake (but you need it to stay calm!). You are told to stop any strenuous exercise, so you stop your sweat-inducing boot camp class, which doesn't make you all that upset. You drink kombucha tea and take herbs that are supposed to promote blood flow. You see an acupuncturist and attempt to relax with needles in your head.

You try to harness the power of that book *The Secret*, not having read it or anything, and visualize happy sperm, voiced by Bruce Willis, swimming with ease up your fallopian tubes. "Go, spermies, go," you sing to them. You eat pineapple because that's what Jennifer the nurse tells you to do. She also tells you there is no scientific evidence behind this.

And each month that you don't get pregnant, you go on a ridiculous drinking bender, which your husband doesn't comment on because, really? C'mon, say something, guy. I dare you.

You consider if perhaps you are just not meant to have a baby. "Plenty of kids need good homes," you say to anyone who wants to hear. You mean it too. They agree, "Of course, of course, there is nothing wrong with adoption." They don't believe it themselves, though. An adopted baby won't have your smile, or your husband's blue eyes, or your love of pickles. But it also won't have your autoimmune disease or your mother's history of depression or your fat ankles, so there's that too.

You wonder, often, if all of this—money, stress, heartache—is even worth it. Babies aren't that great. They are actually a real pain in the ass. And breastfeeding seems weird to you, and poopy diapers are gross. You don't need a baby. You have a career and, more than that, dreams of a bigger career. You are incubating aspirations, and they are almost ready to hatch. You have autonomy and opportunity and perky boobs.

But then you get a call from your nephew on the phone. "Hi Abby! We are eating cookies." And nothing sounds more appealing than sitting around with your own kid, eating cookies on a Sunday afternoon. So you call the IVF nurse and tell her, "Well, Jennifer, I am back at day one, again."

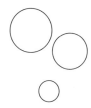

Source Acknowledgments

"By the Numbers" by Melissa Anderson was previously published in *Raw Lit*.

"These Rooms Alone" by Jill Talbot and Marcia Aldrich was previously published in *Longreads*.

"Secrets" by Sari Fordham was previously published in *Pithead Chapel*.

"Notes for the Babysitter" by Lori Sebastianutti was previously published in *Nurture: A Literary Journal*.

"Old Birds and Empty Nests" by Sonya Huber was previously published in *Oldster*.

"The Antidote" by Abigail Thomas was previously published in *Revel*.

"Becoming Your Own Sexual Advocate: A History of Oppression and the Victories Involving Reproductive Rights" by Hillary Leftwich was previously published in *New Skin Magazine*.

"A Story of Two Births" by Jennifer Alessi was previously published in *Mutha Magazine*.

"Monsters" by Aileen Weintraub is an excerpt from *Knocked Down: A High-Risk Memoir* (University of Nebraska Press 2022).

"The Five Stages of Out-of-Place Grief" by Sammi LaBue was previously published in *Sonora Review*.

"Back at Day One Again" by Abby Koenig was previously published in *The Cascadia Subduction Zone*.

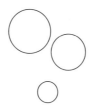

Author Biographies

MARCIA ALDRICH is the author of the free memoir *Girl Rearing*, published by W. W. Norton; *Companion to an Untold Story*, which won the AWP Award for Creative Nonfiction; and *Studio of the Voice*, published by Wandering Aengus Press. She is the editor of *Waveform: Twenty-First-Century Essays by Women*, published by the University of Georgia Press. Her chapbook, *EDGE*, was published by New Michigan Press. Her website is www.marciaaldrich.com.

JENNIFER ALESSI holds a BA in English from Columbia University and an MFA in Creative Writing from the University of Alaska. Her essays have appeared in a dozen publications, including *Hippocampus*, *River Teeth: Beautiful Things*, and *Mutha Magazine*, in which "A Story of Two Births" originally appeared.

MELISSA FLORES ANDERSON is a Latinx Californian and an award-winning journalist who lives in her hometown with her young son and husband. A 2023 Best of the Net nominee for creative nonfiction, her creative work has been published in more than two dozen journals and anthologies, and she is a reader/editor with *Roi Fainéant Press*. *Emerge Literary Journal* included her piece "Layers" in their 2023 anthology *Awakenings:*

Stories of Body and Consciousness and published a coauthored novelette, *Roadkill*, in 2024. Follow her on X and Bluesky @melissacuisine or IG/Threads @theirishmonths. Read her work at www.melissafloresandersonwrites.com.

EMMA BOLDEN is the author of a memoir, *The Tiger and the Cage: A Memoir of a Body in Crisis* (Soft Skull Press, 2022), and the poetry collections *House Is an Enigma* (Southeast Missouri State University Press, 2018), *medi(t)ations* (Noctuary Press, 2016), and *Maleficae* (GenPop Books, 2013). The recipient of a Creative Writing Fellowship from the NEA, her work has appeared in such journals as *Ploughshares*, *The Gettysburg Review*, *New England Review*, *Seneca Review*, *Pleiades*, *Prairie Schooner*, *TriQuarterly*, and *Shenandoah*. She currently serves as an editor of *Screen Door Review: Literary Voices of the Queer South*.

CHLOE CALDWELL is the author of the essay collection *I'll Tell You in Person*, the novella *WOMEN*, and the memoir *The Red Zone: A Love Story*. Her essays have been published in *The New York Times*, *Bon Appétit*, *The Cut*, *The Strategist*, *Longreads*, *The Sun*, and more. Chloe lives in Hudson, New York.

KATIE CLAUSEN's work straddles creative writing, memoir, and academic scholarship. Her writing explores beauty standards deconstruction, fairy tales, feminism, and the transformative power of stories. She holds an MFA in Writing for Children and Young Adults from Simmons University and is currently pursuing a PhD in Information Studies. In 2023, her poem, "holes," won the National Poetry Contest for *Sand Hills Literary Magazine*. Katie currently works as a librarian in the Chicago suburbs.

ARIELLE DANCE, PhD, is an award-winning author who identifies as a Black queer woman with disabilities based in New Jersey. Dr. Dance is published across multiple online platforms and is the author of the award-winning children's book *Dearest One*, which focuses on mindfulness and grief. Most recently, Dr. Dance's manuscript, *Miss Mimi's Welcomes All*, is the second-place winner of the Black Voices in Children's Literature Writing Contest (Free Spirit Publishing).

ANGELIQUE FAWNS is a journalist, author, and television producer. She has a bachelor of journalism degree from Carleton University in Ottawa and almost thirty years of experience as a commercial producer. She's sold more than sixty short stories and is notorious for her submissions blog at www.fawns.ca. Find her scribblings in *Ellery Queen Mystery Magazine*, in *Amazing Stories*, and in her local newspaper.

SARI FORDHAM is a writer, professor, and environmental activist. Her memoir *Wait for God to Notice* narrates her childhood in Uganda. Her work has appeared in *Brevity*, *Best of the Net*, *Booth*, *Baltimore Review*, and *Passages North*, among others. She teaches creative nonfiction at SUNY Oswego and lives in upstate New York with her husband and daughter.

KATEY FUNDERBURGH is a queer Colorado poet. She is a current MFA candidate at George Mason University, where she also teaches courses on composition and literature. Katey serves as a Poetry Alive! fellow and as a co-coordinator for the Incarcerated Writers Program. Some of her other writing appears in *The Blood Pudding*, *Overtly Lit*, and *Pigeon Pages*, among others. When Katey isn't writing, you can find her in the sun with her cat, Thistle. Or find her on X @coloradoKatey.

JULIE HOHULIN lives in Chicago and is a retired marketing professional with a lifelong love of writing. She was first published in *Appalachian Trailway News* in 2004 under the name Julie Ramlo when her essay about walking the Appalachian Trail with her father won first place in the 2003 Trail Days Writing Contest. Since then, Julie has continued to write essays and poetry inspired by her personal experiences as a daughter, wife, mother, and grandmother.

SONYA HUBER is the author of eight books, including the new essay collection *Love and Industry: A Midwestern Workbook* as well as the writing guide *Voice First: A Writer's Manifesto* and an award-winning essay collection on chronic pain, *Pain Woman Takes Your Keys and Other Essays from a Nervous System*. Her other books include *Supremely Tiny Acts: A Memoir in a Day*, *Opa Nobody*, *Cover Me: A Health Insurance Memoir*, and *The Backwards Research Guide for Writers*. Her work has appeared in *The New York Times*, *Brevity*, *Creative Nonfiction*, *The Atlantic*, *The Guardian*, and other outlets. She teaches at Fairfield University and in the Fairfield low-residency MFA program.

ABBY KOENIG has been a writer of all sorts: produced playwright, failed novelist, semi-famous blogger for a minute, something of a journalist, and academic writer with several published journal articles that no one has read. She has directed theater and performed on the stage. She holds a PhD in Rhetoric and Communication and teaches adults many things related to communication. She did eventually get her babies—two at once.

ALYSE KNORR is an associate professor of English at Regis University, co-editor of Switchback Books, and co-producer of the Sweetbitter podcast. She is the author of the poetry collection *Ardor* (2023), a Lambda Literary Award finalist, as well as *Mega-City Redux* (2017), *Copper Mother* (2016), and *Annotated Glass* (2013). She also authored the video game history books *GoldenEye* (2022) and *Super Mario Bros. 3* (2016) and four poetry chapbooks. Her work has appeared or is forthcoming in *The New Republic*, *Poetry Magazine*, *Alaska Quarterly Review*, *Denver Quarterly*, and *The Georgia Review*, among others. She received her MFA from George Mason University.

A Brooklyn-based writer and educator, **SAMMI LABUE** is the founder of Fledgling Writing Workshops (Best Workshop in NYC, *Time Out* 2019), the author of the creative writer's guided journal *Words in Progress* (DK 2020), and basically obsessed with the feeling of having an idea and writing it down. Some of her other nonfiction work can be found in *Literary Hub*, *Glamour*, *The Offing*, *Hobart*, and *Sonora Review*, among others. She received her MFA from the Vermont College of Fine Arts, is *The Penn Review*'s 2024 Poetry Prize winner, and has recently finished a dual memoir written in collaboration with her mom titled *Bad Apples*.

HILLARY LEFTWICH is the author of two books, *Ghosts Are Just Strangers Who Know How to Knock* (Agape Editions, 2023, new edition) and *Aura* (Future Tense Books and Blackstone Audio Publishing, 2022). She owns Alchemy Author Services and Writing Workshop and teaches writing at several universities and colleges along with Lighthouse Writers, a local nonprofit for adults and youth. Her latest work can be found or is forthcoming in *The Sun*, *Santa Fe Writers Project*, and *The Rumpus*. She lives in Denver, Colorado.

DEBORAH MELTVEDT is a writer and health educator in Sacramento, California. She loves blending poetry and creative nonfiction with medical themes. Deborah taught reproductive health, mental health, and global health studies in public high schools for many years. She has been published in various literary and medical anthologies, and her first book of poetry, *Becoming a Woman*, was published by the Poetry Box in 2021. Currently a volunteer at a local Planned Parenthood clinic, Deborah lives with her husband, Rick, and their cat, Anchovy Jack.

LEAH MUELLER's work appears in *Rattle*, *NonBinary Review*, *Brilliant Flash Fiction*, *The Citron Review*, *The Spectacle*, *New Flash Fiction Review*, *Atticus Review*, *Your Impossible Voice*, and more. She has been nominated for Pushcart and Best of the Net prizes. Leah appears in the 2022 edition of *Best Small Fictions*. Her fourteenth book, *Stealing Buddha*, was published by Anxiety Press in 2024. Her website is www.leahmueller.org.

YODA OLINYK loves to make people comfortable, which is too bad because she is a writer. Yoda believes creativity is a chance to reveal the sharp corners of life and writes mostly about addiction and grief; she is currently working on a book about abortion in Canada. Yoda's poems have been published with *Button Poetry*, *samfiftyfour*, *Third Iris*, *Sky Island Journal*, *Free Verse*, *Ink & Marrow*, *Sage Cigarettes*, and *Quail Bell*. Yoda works full time as a writing coach and book doula and also wrote a full-length, best-selling memoir called *Salt & Sour*. You can find more of Yoda's work at www.doulaofwords.com.

MONICA PRINCE teaches activist and performance writing and serves as the Director of Africana Studies at Susquehanna University. She's the author of several collections, including

Roadmap: A Choreopoem and *How to Exterminate the Black Woman*. As the foremost choreopoem scholar, she writes, performs, and directs choreopoems across the country.

LORI SEBASTIANUTTI is a writer and teacher from Ontario, Canada. Her essays have been published in Canadian and American journals, including *Hamilton Review of Books*, *The Humber Literary Review*, *The New Quarterly*, *Nurture*, *Porcupine Literary*, *Serotonin*, and *Broadview*, among others. Her award-winning essay "Cutting Ties and Letting Go" is forthcoming in *An Anthology of Canadian Birth Stories*, published by Praeclarus Press.

SARAH SWANDELL is a writer and pastor whose work has appeared in *The Christian Century*, *100 Word Story*, *Coffee + Crumbs*, and *Journal of Compressed Creative Arts*. Find her at www.sarahswandell.com.

JILL TALBOT is the author of *The Last Year: Essays*, winner of the Wandering Aengus Editor's Prize, as well as *The Way We Weren't: A Memoir* and *Loaded: Women and Addiction*. *A Distant Town: Stories* won the 2021 Jeanne Leiby Memorial Chapbook Contest and was published by *The Florida Review*. Her essays have appeared in *AGNI*, *Brevity*, *Gulf Coast*, *Hotel Amerika*, *LitMag*, *River Teeth*, *Southwest Review*, *The Rumpus*, and *The Paris Review Daily*, among others. She is an associate professor and University Distinguished Teaching Professor at University of North Texas.

ABIGAIL THOMAS has written two short story collections, one novel, four memoirs, a book on how to write memoir called *Thinking About Memoir*, and three children's books. She has four children, twelve grandchildren, two great-grandchildren, and a high school education. Her most recent book is *Still Life at Eighty:*

The Next Interesting Thing. She is working on a tiny book about making things out of clay, and she lives with her two dogs in Woodstock, New York.

STEPHANIE VESSELY holds an MFA in Creative Writing from Regis University and is currently seeking publication for her essay collection, which was longlisted in the Santa Fe Writers Project Literary Awards. Her work appears in *December Magazine*, *Hippocampus Magazine*, *The Offing*, and elsewhere, and has been nominated for a Pushcart Prize. Find her at www.stephanievessely.com or on X and Instagram @vesselywriter.

JOY VICTORY is an editor and writer based in Austin, Texas. Her newsletter, *The Shrieking Cactus*, delves into overcoming midlife trauma and learning to be less prickly in life. Her work has appeared in *Texas Monthly*, *The Sun*, *Dorothy Parker's Ashes*, *San Antonio Review*, *VICE*, and *Cosmopolitan*. She's also revising a memoir about the impact of her mother's severe mental illness on her own mental health, interwoven with stories of the resilient wildlife of South Texas.

AILEEN WEINTRAUB is a memoirist whose book *Knocked Down: A High-Risk Memoir* is a University of Nebraska Press bestseller and a journalist whose work has been featured in *Oprah Daily*, *The Washington Post*, *BBC*, *Huff Post*, and many others. She is also an award-winning children's book author. You can find out more about her at www.aileenweintraub.com.